Dr. Doctor's
Little Back Book

**All the secrets you need to know about causes and
solutions for neck, mid-back, and lower back pain**

Uday Doctor, M.D.

REVIEWS OF DR. DOCTOR'S LITTLE BACK BOOK

"*Dr. Doctor's Little Back Book* is a must-read for the person with back or neck pain looking for an answer. The book enables patients with spine pain to play an important role in their own diagnosis and treatment. Dr. Doctor's unique diagnose and then treat approach is a complete reversal of how most pain is managed currently, which is usually to treat the symptoms with no endpoint. He has found a way to almost eliminate the use of narcotics in the treatment of spine pain. Dr. Doctor's techniques described in this book have been proven successful in everyone from the professional athlete to the weekend golfer. *Dr. Doctor's Little Back Book* is meant to be flexible, useful, and handy. Patients want resources they understand and can use."

Walter R. Lowe, *M.D.*,
Edward T. Smith Endowed Chair of Department of Orthopedic Surgery,
University of Texas Medical School, Houston, Head Physician for NFL Houston
Texans, NBA Houston Rockets, and NCAA University of Houston Cougars

"Dr. Doctor has provided the Houston Astros with excellent medical care and assisted us greatly with keeping our players on the field during our 2017 World Series Championship season. It comes as no surprise that he has put together an excellent book appropriate for everyone who has neck or back pain. Not only does he thoroughly explain common back issues in detail, but he provides simple treatment fixes that help alleviate symptoms and pain. Highly recommend for anyone with acute or chronic back pain."

Jeremiah Randall, *P.T., D.P.T., A.T.C., C.S.C.S., Certified D.N.*,
Head Athletic Trainer and Physical Therapist for
MLB 2017 World Series Champions Houston Astros

"Highly recommend *Dr. Doctor's Little Back Book*, whether you have back or neck pain, or are a physician, physical therapist, or other allied health-care provider. This book is appropriate for all populations, whether you are a weekend warrior or a hurting patient. The *Little Back Book* covers the same unique approach that Dr. Doctor uses to diagnose and treat back pain in professional athletes, and his **Straight Spine Safe Spine** Therapy and Exercise Program shows how invaluable body positions, posture, and the right exercises are to prevent back and neck pain for everybody."

Geoff Kaplan, *A.T.C., P.T., S.C.S., C.S.C.S.*,
Director of Sports Medicine and Head
Athletic Trainer for NFL Houston Texans

"*Dr. Doctor's Little Back Book* provides clear direction to navigate the complex world of back pain. He describes a comprehensive system that provides a more purposeful approach to diagnosing and treating spine pathology in order to optimize a patient's outcome and function."

Jason Biles, *D.P.T., A.T.C., S.C.S.,*
Head Athletic Trainer for NBA Houston Rockets

"Dr. Doctor is an incredible diagnostician and technically outstanding at what he does. The *Little Back Book* is a reflection of his expertise. This is a gem for all patients who suffer from spinal pathology and go down the treatment pathway. The *Little Back Book* is truly original in its form of being directed at educating patients about their problem, the clinical manifestations, and treatments available. It will likely help many patients as Dr. Doctor has done in his many years in practice."

Mark L. Prasarn, *M.D.,*
Chief, Division of Spine Surgery, Department of Orthopedic Surgery, University of Texas, Houston, Spine Consultant for NBA Houston Rockets, Assistant Team Physician for NFL Houston Texans

"Dr. Doctor is the main reason that I am coaching into my 80's. Dr. Doctor's dedication to and knowledge of problems of the spine as described in the *Little Back Book* makes this book unique. This book should be the bible for spine care."

Wayne Graham,
Head Baseball Coach,
Rice University, Houston, Texas

"He is, without a doubt, one of the most knowledgeable physicians on the planet in regard to the diagnosis and treatment of spine pain. This book will help all patients who read it, and it is also a valuable resource for health-care providers who seek straightforward education and answers to the most important issues in managing pain that arises from the spine."

David S. Baskin, *M.D., F.A.C.S., F.A.A.N.S.,*
Kenneth R. Peak Presidential Distinguished Chair,
Vice Chair and Residency Program Director, Department of Neurosurgery, Houston Methodist Hospital,
Professor of Neurosurgery, Weill Cornell Medical College

"The treatment and exercises that Dr. Doctor illustrates in the *Little Back Book* are the same ones he has used to keep college athletes on the field. I would strongly urge anyone with back or neck pain to read this book!"

David Pierce,
Head Baseball Coach,
University of Texas, Austin

"My first impression of Dr. Doctor was that I couldn't believe a dude wearing cowboy boots with his scrubs was actually going to take care of my pain issue! The *Little Back Book* is a reflection of him and how simply he solves back pain. His explanation and solution was right to the point and so is his book, which is self-explanatory and easy to follow."

Kelvin Sampson,
Head Basketball Coach,
University of Houston, Texas

Uday Doctor, M.D.
U Doctor Medical PLLC
Fondren Orthopedic Group LLP
7401 Main Street
Houston, TX 77030

www.straightspinesafespine.com

Illustrated by Beth Sumner, M.A., C.M.I., and
jehsomwang © 123rf.com (cover cartoon and select works)

Medical Editorial Panel:

David Lintner, *M.D., Chief, Sports Medicine and Fellowship Director, Houston Methodist Hospital, Head Physician for MLB Houston Astros, Team Orthopedist for NFL Houston Texans*

David Wimberley, *M.D., Spine Surgeon, Fondren Orthopedic Group, Texas Orthopedic Hospital*

Mark L. Prasarn, *M.D., Chief, Division of Spine Surgery, Department of Orthopedic Surgery, University of Texas, Houston, Spine Consultant for NBA Houston Rockets, Assistant Team Physician for NFL Houston Texans*

Walter R. Lowe, *M.D., Edward T. Smith Endowed Chair of Department of Orthopedic Surgery, University of Texas Medical School, Houston, Head Physician for NFL Houston Texans, NBA Houston Rockets, and NCAA University of Houston Cougars*

Printed in the United States of America.

First Edition

ISBN: 978-1-7321339-0-7

This book is dedicated to all my past and present patients as well as to my wife, Nancy, and children, Emily and William, whose patience and support were greatly appreciated during the five years that it took to make this book come to fruition.

Dr. Doctor's Little Back Book

All the secrets you need to know about causes and solutions for neck, mid-back, and lower back pain

Uday Doctor, M.D.

Table of Contents

Foreword

Pain is probably the world's oldest medical problem and the most universal affliction of humankind, and yet very little is known about its basic mechanisms and how to best treat it. The ancient Greeks regarded pain as an external force, which entered the body through a wound and slowly worked to destroy it. One of the earliest concepts of pain can be found in the Book of Genesis, in which pain was a source of punishment from God for sin and evil activity. When Eve fell from grace, God told her to expect more pain.

Despite many centuries of firsthand experience with pain and its many potential treatments, even technology today frequently fails both to properly diagnose pain and its causes and to guide treatment. In particular, lower back pain and neck pain are the most common disabilities in the United States today. Americans miss more days from work because of these conditions than because of the three biggest killers, namely, cancer, stroke, and heart disease.

The result is an incredibly confusing state for patients with spine pain. How does one gain an understanding of one's painful condition and what causes it? More importantly, what is the best course to take to alleviate and reduce the devastating effects of pain on patients, families, communities, and society as a whole?

Sir Francis Bacon once wrote that knowledge is power, and this wonderful book explains the anatomy and causes of spine pain and state-of-the-art treatments in a straightforward, highly accurate, and easily understandable way.

Uday Doctor, M.D., guides the reader through a crystal-clear journey that unravels the many mysteries of back pain and its treatment. He starts with easy-to-understand and concise descriptions of the anatomy of the spine and its nerves, explaining how abnormalities produce pain. He then discusses alternative treatments, therapies, exercises, and medications that can be used to manage spine pain. Drawing on his vast experience for more than twenty years performing thousands of these procedures skillfully, he then goes on to describe specific minimally invasive diagnostic and potentially therapeutic procedures specific to each type of problem. He clearly explains the role of whole-body exercises and the importance of specific proper body mechanics that can minimize pain and prevent recurrences. Finally, he ends with a common-sense and straightforward set of answers to questions asked by many patients with pain.

I have personally worked with Uday Doctor for more than twenty years helping patients with pain, and he is, without a doubt, one of the most knowledgeable physicians on the planet in regard to the diagnosis and treatment of spine pain. This book will help all patients who read it, and it is also a valuable resource for health-care providers who seek straightforward education and answers to the most important issues in managing pain that arises from the spine.

David S. Baskin, M.D., F.A.C.S., F.A.A.N.S.
Kenneth R. Peak Presidential Distinguished Chair; Vice Chair and Residency Program Director, Department of Neurosurgery, Houston Methodist Hospital; Senior Member, Houston Methodist Research Institute; Professor of Neurosurgery, Weill Cornell Medical College; Professor of Engineering and Research Professor of Pharmacy, University of Houston; Director, Kenneth R. Peak Brain and Pituitary Tumor Treatment Center

Preface

I have spent the last twenty years diagnosing and treating all types of pain that originate from the spine, everything from neck pain all the way down to a pain in the butt. I decided to write this book at the urging of a lot of my patients who came to see me with many questions and even more "answers." In this era of pain management, laser spine surgery, multiple types of spine therapy, and unlimited information on the Internet, patients have a hard time deciding what to do, as they consider whether the answers available to them are true!

Between the television ads proclaiming the latest miracle back cures, the enlightenment of computer advertising on the quick fix for back pain, and medical practitioners relying on the latest scan or test that would tell them the exact diagnosis for their patient's spine pain, it occurred to me that the most common-sense and basic knowledge that people need to know about their spine has now become almost a "secret," like you would find in a little black book. Or more appropriately the *Little Back Book*. I finally decided that it was time to share some information as well as answer many of the questions that I am asked every day.

The questions that I have been asked involve a wide variety of topics. Patients ask the simple question of why their neck or back hurts and then want to know which exercises they need to do so their pain will not return. Some come to the office unable to sit on their tailbone and wonder why, while others are puzzled why the therapy that they were doing for their back or neck pain created more pain. Some patients could not walk to their mailbox without hurting and asked why it felt so good to sit down or walk bent over. Others could not understand why they could walk all day but could not sit still without squirming due to back pain. I have had patients who noticed pain in their ribs when they bent forward or twisted, and others who felt like there was a knife in their shoulder blade.

A lot of these patients had been treated without ever locating the specific structure that was creating their discomfort. Some of them had endured therapy, multiple injections, and even surgery without ever identifying the exact problem that was creating their pain. Many of these same patients had been given the "chronic pain" label and placed on narcotics without ever reaching a diagnosis. There is an epidemic in this country because of the liberal use of narcotics to treat "pain" as a diagnosis instead of a symptom that needs a diagnosis.

This book is based on one premise: *identify the problem and then treat it.* If you first locate the problem that is creating your pain, you can then do the right therapy, obtain the right injections, perform the right exercises, and, if needed, have the correct surgical operation for your specific problem. You will see very early in this book that this premise does not mean just to obtain an MRI of the painful area. The MRI shows only the wear and tear, but it does *not* show pain. You may have a tear in your rotator cuff, but the pain in your shoulder could be coming from your spine. Or you may have a very degenerated hip joint, but the pain in your hip could be coming from your spine. What you will see in this book is that I wrote most of the chapters based on patients' complaints. I am going to show you how to use your own information about your pain to help you find out why you hurt.

This book will educate you about your spine, help you find out why you hurt, show you alternatives on how to treat your pain, and finally, point out how learning about body mechanics and exercise can help prevent recurrences of pain. Use this book as only one source of information, as you will discover many ways to take care of spine pain. But, if you remember only one thing from this book, it is this: *diagnose* and *then* treat.

Uday Doctor, M.D.
Chief, Spinal Diagnostics and Therapeutics Division,
Texas Orthopedic Hospital, Houston

A Note to the Readers of This Book

This book was written to be a helpful source of information for anyone who has ever had back or neck pain, or pain in other areas of the body that may be due to the spine, such as arm, leg, shoulder, hip, buttock, and groin. The content of this book comes not only from my personal experience of diagnosing and treating patients over the last twenty years, but also from what I have learned while dealing with my own back and neck pain over an even longer period of time. I have to credit numerous spine surgeons and neurosurgeons who led me in the direction of diagnosing spine pain prior to treatment, instead of just managing the symptoms. I must also thank all my patients, as I learned that the secret to diagnosing back or neck pain rests in the information that the patients possess about their pain, instead of in an MRI or other tests.

This book should be used only as one source of information to help you understand your back or neck pain and should not be a replacement for a health-care practitioner. I hope that this book would be used in conjunction with your health-care professional, whether a physician, chiropractor, or physical therapist.

How to Use This Book

I suggest you use this book by first reading the three chapters in Part I. This section will provide you with a basic understanding of your spine and show you why it is important to locate the specific problem that may be creating your pain.

Then read all the chapters that pertain to your pain in Part II (Chapters 4–14). Note, however, that this book is primarily about pain that originates from the spine and joints, so do not think of it as a complete medical book. For example, if you have groin pain, it could come from a hernia or another medical problem. If everything else has been ruled out and you are not getting better, then you should read the chapter on groin pain. You also will notice that I wrote each of these chapters based on one specific complaint that patients have about their pain or one specific area of the body that hurts. For example, one chapter deals with back and leg pain when you walk and another chapter discusses back pain when you sit. There is a chapter on buttock pain and another one on hip pain. The reason I did this is that patients usually have one major complaint or area that is bothering them when they come to see me. They tell me just that *either something specific creates their pain or one specific area hurts*. You may notice that more than one chapter pertains to your pain. For example, your hip may hurt and you have back and leg pain when you walk. Or your arm and your shoulder blade hurt. A lot of the problems in the spine can and usually do create pain in different areas of the body at the same time. For example, the lumbar nerve in your back can create pain in the buttock, groin, and leg all at the same time, or the pain can be isolated in just the leg or buttock.

Read every chapter that pertains to your area of pain. If your back and leg pain get worse if you walk or sit, you should read both Chapters 4 and 6. You may notice a lot of repetition of pictures, comments, and ideas in different chapters. Most people will go directly to the chapter that pertains to their specific area of pain and then look for answers in the rest of the book. Therefore, I touch on things that I mention in the first three chapters throughout the rest of the book.

You can finish by reading Part III. Chapters 15 to 17 give you alternatives for treatment, therapy, and exercises. Chapter 15 discusses different medications that can be used for managing the pain. Chapter 16 goes over specific minimally invasive diagnostic procedures to diagnose and treat the specific problem that may be creating your pain.

Chapter 17 will introduce you to the **Straight Spine Safe Spine** Program, which provides specific exercises and therapy for each part of the spine that may be creating your pain. The **Straight Spine Safe Spine** Program will also teach you how to live your daily life using proper body mechanics and ergonomics, as well as explain how to exercise so that the least amount of stress is placed on your spine.

Chapter 18 lists the most common questions that I am asked every day regarding spine pain. The answers to these questions are based on my experience over the last twenty years, and they should be considered just as one source of information, since there are many different views when it comes to spine pain.

PART I

The Spine and How It Creates Pain

Introduction to the Diagnose and Treat Method

Even though a lot of information is available to the public regarding the general diagnosis and treatment of back pain, and many different medical practitioners deal with spine pain, I continue to see patients who show up in my office, hurting, without a specific diagnosis. They may already have had a lot of MRIs, physical therapy, injections, surgery, and other forms of care, but the biggest problem facing most of these patients is that they do not have a *specific diagnosis.*

The proper way to treat any medical problem is to *find* the exact cause of the problem and then attempt to *fix it.* When it comes to spine pain—whether it is neck or back pain, or some form of pain that runs down the arm, leg, hip, or shoulder that is created by the spine—I have noticed that instead of locating the specific problem in the spine and then finding a way to eliminate it, the usual medical care is to treat every back and neck problem the same way. This may be the *same* type of physical therapy, the *same* type of exercise program, and/or the *same* type of injections. You will find that as you read this book, depending on the exact structure in the spine that is creating your pain, the therapy, the injections, and your exercise program can be completely different. I see patients all the time for whom *one* essential issue has not been resolved: *they do not have a specific diagnosis!*

Okay, I know I am repeating myself, but this is an important point that I am always trying to get across to patients and other medical practitioners. You may be wondering why there could be an issue like this with all the technology that now exists. Why not just get an MRI of the area that is creating your pain, find the inflamed area on the MRI that is creating your pain, and then treat it? I am going to discuss this in detail later in this chapter, but the simple answer to that question is that an MRI just shows wear and tear and not pain. And we all have wear and tear as we age. Most people will go through their life with herniated discs and arthritic joints in their spine with no pain. The only time you are usually going to hurt is when the disc, the nerve, or the joint becomes inflamed, and the MRI does not show inflammation. You cannot make a diagnosis by just obtaining an MRI.

The care of the spine that is discussed in this book rests on one simple premise: **diagnose first and then treat**.

Actually, the first step isn't diagnosis at all. The reality is that eighty percent of all people with acute back or neck pain will get better over a period of weeks with no medical treatment at all—because the body will heal itself by eliminating the inflammation. Many people during their lifetime are going to have neck, mid-back, or lower back pain because of poor body mechanics or a specific twisting turning motion that tweaked the disc, nerve, or joint. This pain is usually due to a disc, nerve, and/or joint in the spine that becomes red, hot, swollen, and painful as the body reacts to the injury. The swelling and pain go away over several weeks as the body goes to work eliminating this inflammation. Therefore, it is not necessary to find a specific reason for your pain during the first several weeks, because your pain will probably resolve no matter what is done. The only reason not to treat your pain conservatively during the first month or so is if you have severe numbness or weakness in your arms or legs or if the pain is not controlled by oral medications.

What this means is that if you have an acute attack of back or neck pain, just try to treat it with your favorite combination of anti-inflammatory drugs, ice, heat, and pain medication, and try to stay as active as possible without creating excess pain. You need to wait it out and see whether you are going to be one of the eighty percent who will get better without doing anything else. If you want to see your local chiropractor or physical therapist, go right ahead, as these practitioners can be helpful during this period. The information on therapy and exercises in Chapter 17 can be used in conjunction with your therapist or chiropractor, but during this period, do *not* do any specific exercises that create pain. The body is trying to tell you something. Listen to it.

Do not get caught up with a lot of medical mumbo-jumbo during this time. You may hear that you need multiple days of traction, a series of injections, realignment of your hips, and maybe even a surgery or two. Ignore this advice at this time. Also, forget the running, weight lifting, yoga, and anything else that involves twisting and pounding of your spine. This is a period of healing. Once the pain gets better, skip down to Chapter 17 in this book and go from there. I put this chapter at the end of the book for a reason. Most patients are able to exercise much better *after* their acute pain is gone and they know specifically what is creating their pain. So even though you may be able to use some of these exercises during your acute pain, the most beneficial time is after you are feeling better. What I am telling you is that no matter what area in your spine is creating the pain, most of the time the body will eradicate the inflammation. A diagnosis is not important during the first several weeks of your pain unless you are having significant numbness or weakness.

If your discomfort persists after four to six weeks, then it is time to read the rest of this book. The first thing you need to do is to locate where your pain is coming from. You can start by marking the areas where you feel the discomfort on an outline of the human body. I am going to show you an illustration of the front and back of the human body, which is called a pain diagram (**Picture 1**). It allows patients to draw on it to show the exact area where they feel their discomfort. I have patients complete this drawing before I see them. So if you are hurting at this time, you can draw where your pain is located on this image.

You may be wondering why I am asking you to draw on a picture before telling you anything about the spine. The answer is that this is the most important "secret" piece of information that you will want to read about in this whole book! Just matching your pain drawing with *three* pictures, **Picture 2**, **Picture 3**, and **Picture 5**, which show where structures in the spine create pain, will enable you to narrow down the problem that is creating your pain.

The next picture that I am going to show you is a front and back picture of the human body that specifically shows the different areas where you will feel pain on the surface of the body when the nerves in the spine are inflamed (Picture 2).

You will see a letter and a number attached to each area. The neck is called the cervical area, the mid-back is the thoracic area, and the lower back is the lumbar area. Therefore, a C in front of the number corresponds to the cervical or neck area, the T stands for mid-back or thoracic area, and the L stands for the lumbar or lower back. The S in the picture refers to the sacral or tailbone area. The number attached to the letter gives the specific nerve. For example, C6 stands for the sixth cervical nerve, the L5 nerve is the fifth lumbar nerve, and T10 stands for the tenth thoracic nerve. If you follow each one of these nerves, you will see that each has a specific path. The cervical nerves start in the neck and go down into the shoulders and arms. The thoracic nerves start in the mid-back and wrap all the way around to the front of the body. The lumbar nerves start in the lower back and go down the front and back of the legs. The sacral nerves primarily cover the pelvic area.

If you drew on the pain diagram in Picture 1, you can now match it to Picture 2. For example, if you drew your pain on the side or back of the leg, it would match L4, L5, or S1. If you drew your pain in the area of the shoulder blade, it would match T4 or T5. If you drew your pain over the hip, it would match the L4 or L5 nerve. If you drew over the back of the neck, it would match C5, C6, C7, or C8. Remember that Picture 2 points out only where the nerves in the spine create pain on the surface of the body. You should keep in mind other possibilities. The first is that the problem could be with a joint or muscle, and not the spine. So, if your shoulder hurts, your pain could be

Pain Diagram
Mark the areas on your body where you feel the
described sensations. Use appropriate symbol.
Mark areas of radiation.
Include all affected areas.

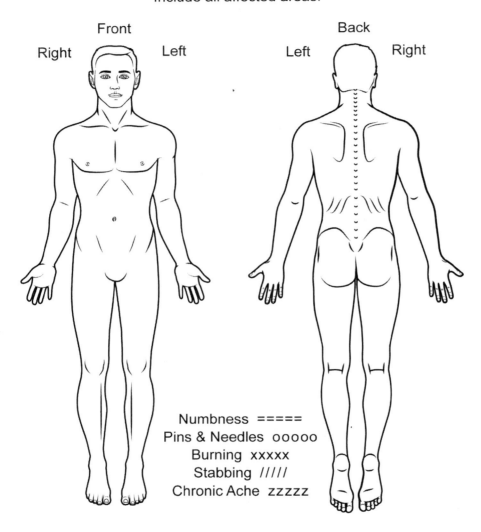

Numbness =====
Pins & Needles ooooo
Burning xxxxx
Stabbing /////
Chronic Ache zzzzz

Estimate the severity of your pain (Choose one number)

0 No Pain
1 Mild Pain
2-3 Moderate Pain

4-5 Moderate to Severe Pain
6-7 Severe Pain
8-9 Intensely Severe Pain
10 Most Severe Pain

PICTURE 1

Pain diagram.

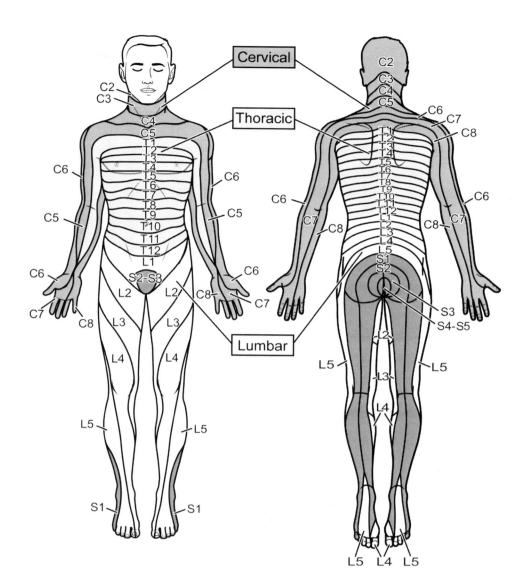

PICTURE 2

This picture shows where the nerves in the spine create pain on the surface of the body when they are inflamed.

coming from your shoulder joint, the muscles around the shoulder, or the nerves that run from your spine to your shoulder, which would be the C5 or C6 nerves. If your knee hurts, the knee joint could be inflamed, or the L3 or L4 nerve root could be causing the pain. If your hip hurts, it could be the hip joint, one of the muscles surrounding the hip joint, or the L4 or L5 nerves creating your pain. The chapters in Part II in this book will help you find the specific source of your pain, but right now just focus on narrowing down the level if the pain is from your spine.

There is another thing that I need to bring up to help you locate the problem that is creating your pain. Remember that I said there were *three* pictures that you had to compare your pain diagram (Picture 1) to? Picture 2, the *first* of the three, showed where you would feel pain over the surface of the body when the nerves are inflamed. These same nerves also go to specific *muscles* and *bones* in the body, and some do not follow the same path as Picture 2. Picture 3 is the *second* picture that you need to look at in order to identify the *muscles* and *bones* in the upper part of the body that may be painful when the nerves in the cervical spine are inflamed.

This picture points out the muscle areas that will hurt when the specific nerve is inflamed. For example, if the C2 or C3 nerve is inflamed, it will create pain in your skull. If the C6 or C7 nerve is inflamed, then you may have pain in the back of your shoulder or the front of your chest. The two areas that I want to point out in Picture 3 because they do not match Picture 2 are the areas of the shoulder blade and the front of the chest, which are covered by the muscles that the C6 and C7 nerves go to. If you had pain in your shoulder blade or in the front of the chest and only looked at Picture 2, you might think that your pain could come only from the thoracic nerves. When you also look at Picture 3, which shows you where the *muscles* and *bones* hurt when the cervical nerves are inflamed, you then can consider the possibility that your pain is coming from the C6 or C7 nerve as well. You should always look at both these pictures together when considering your diagnosis of your upper body.

Picture 4 is a pain drawing from a patient who came in to see me with pain in the back of the shoulder blade, in the front of the chest, and going down the arm to the fingers.

As you can see from this drawing, the areas marked are a combination of Pictures 2 and 3 showing the areas where you could hurt if the C7 nerve is inflamed. Picture 2 did not show the pain from the C7 nerve going all the way down the shoulder blade or to the front of the chest. Picture 3 does. If your shoulder blade hurts and you matched your information just with Picture 2 instead of both Pictures 2 and 3, you would think your pain was coming from T5 or T6. If I had then treated the T5 or T6 nerve and your pain

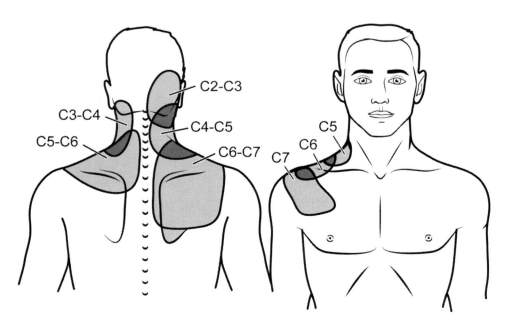

PICTURE 3

Muscles that hurt when specific nerves in the cervical spine are inflamed.

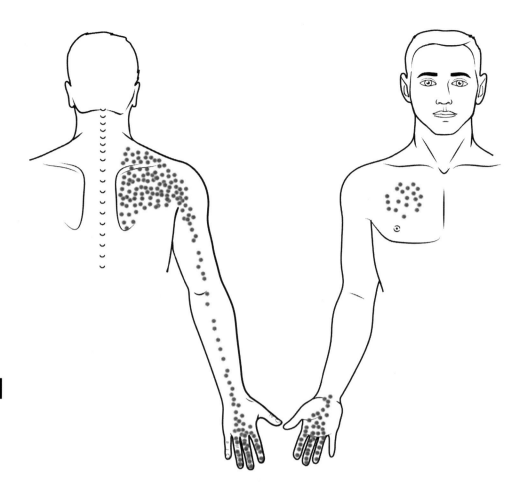

PICTURE 4

Areas of the body where you may feel pain when the C7 nerve is inflamed.

was coming from the C7 nerve, you would not have gotten better. I want to make sure that you understand why you need to look at both pictures. An important thing to remember is that you may *not* have pain in *all* the areas at the same time. For example, if your C7 nerve is inflamed, you could have pain just in the area of the shoulder blade, or pain only going down the arm, or neck pain with no arm or shoulder blade pain, or even just chest pain.

The *third* of the three pictures I mentioned above (Picture 5) shows where inflamed nerves in the lumbar spine create pain in the *muscles* and *bones* of the lower portion of the body, just as Picture 3 shows the same for the cervical spine and the upper body.

We have already examined Picture 2, which shows the area of the surface of the body that may feel pain when the lumbar nerve roots are inflamed. You have to combine Pictures 2 and 5 to be able to fully see where the lumbar nerves create pain. Let me pick out the most common areas in the lower part of the body that patients indicate on their pain diagrams and point out the possible nerves in the spine that could be involved in creating *muscle* and *bone* pain.

The first example I want to point out is the area of the groin on the pain diagram. If you look at Picture 2, it shows that the surface of the groin area is covered by T12, L1, L2, or possibly S1 or S2. When you look at the front of the body in Picture 5, you see that L3, L4, L5, and S1 cover the *muscles* and *bones* of the groin. Remember, your groin may hurt for reasons that have nothing to do with your spine, like a hernia or an arthritic hip, *but* if the pain *is* coming from your spine, it could be coming from any of the lumbar nerves. I am going to talk about groin pain in another chapter, so all I want you to understand now is that when you draw on a pain diagram in the groin area, your pain could be coming from one of the many different nerves in the lumbar spine.

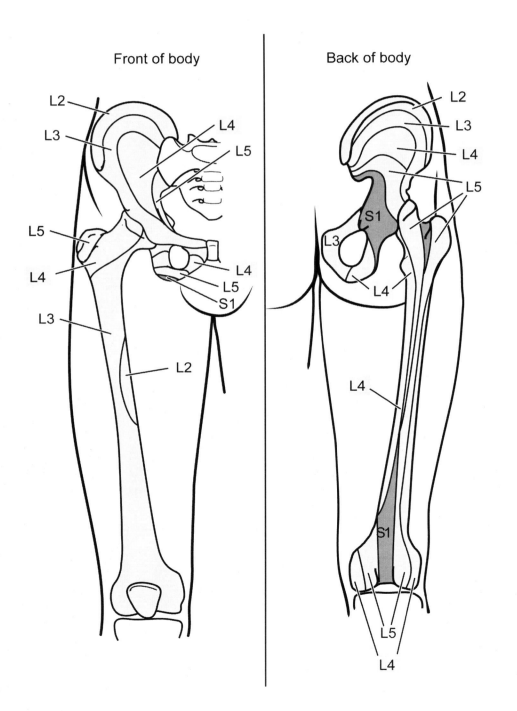

PICTURE 5

Inflamed nerves in the lumbar spine create pain in the muscles and bones of the hip, buttock, and groin.

The next example is the side of your hip. If you look at Picture 2, you will see that L3, L4, and L5 cover the surface of the side of your hip. If you look at the front of the body in Picture 5, you see that the *muscles* and *bones* of the bursa of the hip are covered by the L4 and L5 nerves. I see a lot of patients who come into the office with agonizing pain in the side of the hip area, and they think they have a problem with their hip or the hip bursa. However, most of these patients hurt on the side of the hip because their L4 or L5 nerve is inflamed and *not* because of a bursitis of the hip. You need to treat the L4 and L5 nerves to get better, not the hip bursa. Chapter 7 will help you diagnose your hip pain.

Let me address one more example that I see patients draw on pain diagrams: the buttock area. Picture 2 shows that the S1, S2, and L5 nerves cover the *surface* of the buttock, and Picture 5 shows that the *muscles* and *bones* of the buttock can be covered by L3, L4, L5, and S1. I call attention to this area because many of the patients who consult me about buttock pain have been diagnosed with things like sacroiliac joint pain, hamstring pulls, and even a problem with their piriformis muscle, which is a muscle in the buttock area, when really a nerve in their back is creating their pain.

Picture 6 is a pain diagram illustrating the fifth lumbar nerve (L5), which is one of the most common nerves that become inflamed in the lumbar spine. You will see that it is a combination of Pictures 2 and 5. This nerve travels to several areas, including the hip, back, groin, buttock, and many places on the leg. Picture 2 did not show the L5 nerve going to the groin or deep into the buttock, the two areas that are shown in Picture 5. You may *not* have pain in all the areas shown in Picture 6 at the same time where your L5 nerve is inflamed. You may notice only back pain, or only pain in the foot or hip, or even just pain into the buttock.

I will keep showing you these pictures because they illustrate the most important part of this book. If I can get just one piece of information across to my readers, it would be to understand the concept that nerves in the body can refer pain to multiple areas and that pain can occur far from where the nerve starts. So a nerve in your neck can actually create horrible pain in your shoulder blade or make your fingers numb. A nerve in your back can create pain in your groin, hip, or leg or just make your toes go numb. I refer to Pictures 2, 3, and 5 every day in my practice. I combine the pictures of the *surface of the body* and the *muscles* and *bones* together to get the full explanation. For example, if you have pain in the area of the shoulder blade and I looked at Pictures 2 and 3, I would know that your pain may be coming from the spine, either from the C6 or C7 nerve or T5 or T6. If your buttock hurts, and I look at Pictures 2 and 5, I would then know that your pain could be coming from the L3, L4, L5, or S1 nerves.

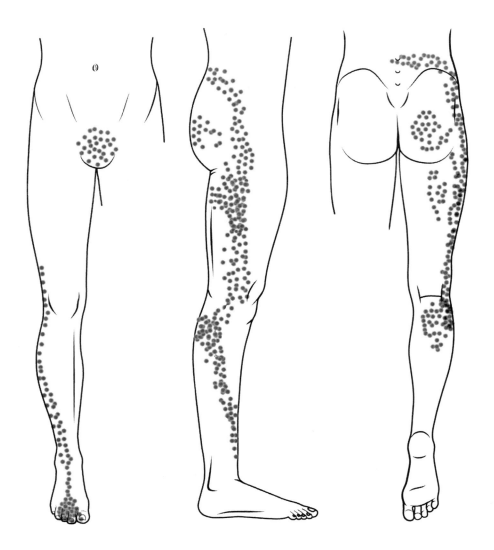

PICTURE 6

The areas of the body where you may feel pain when the L5 nerve is inflamed.

I am not suggesting that all your pain comes from your spine. If you have pain in your shoulder blade area, you do not want to jump to the conclusion that it is coming from your neck (otherwise known as the cervical spine). Just because one of the nerves in the neck goes to your shoulder, this does not mean that your shoulder pain always comes from the neck. The source actually could be your shoulder. If you have pain in your groin, you do not want to automatically decide that it is coming from the L1 nerve. The groin pain could be from some of the other lumbar nerves, a hernia, or even the hip, as the hip creates pain in the area of the groin. Pain in the side of your hip could very well be coming from the L4 and L5 nerves instead of the hip. Pain in your foot could indicate something wrong with your foot and *not* your back. The therapy and treatment for a problem in your spine may be very different from the therapy and treatment for the shoulder or hip.

In the rest of this book, I will take the information from the pain diagram and combine it with a specific history about your pain to help you come up with an answer. The information that *you* know about yourself as it relates to your pain is more important than anything else. What makes your pain worse? What makes your pain better? Does it get worse when you walk? Does looking up or down make your neck hurt? Does your back or neck feel better after a night of rest or is it worse in the morning? The combining of this information, along with your physical exam, should narrow the possibilities of what specific structure is creating the pain, even before you obtain an MRI.

In fact, let's talk about the MRI for a minute. I mentioned earlier in this chapter that an MRI only shows you areas of *degeneration*. Wear and tear. Not pain. Most people over the age of fifty will have degenerated discs, arthritic joints, and compressed nerves—but little pain. What this tells us is that the human body puts up with a lot of degeneration until something really gets inflamed. And as I told you earlier in this chapter, most inflammation subsides on its own as the body takes care of itself. The herniated disc or the arthritis is still there—it's just not inflamed!

> **Remember: The MRI shows degeneration, not where pain is coming from.**

So to find the problem that is creating your pain, you need to match *your* specific information with the MRI to help make a diagnosis. The MRI alone won't be enough.

Let me give you a couple of examples based on the cases mentioned earlier. Let's say that you have shoulder blade pain and had an MRI of the shoulder and the cervical spine. The MRI of the shoulder shows degeneration of the shoulder and the MRI of the neck shows multiple herniated discs. Which should the doctor treat? The shoulder? The cervical spine? Which disc in the neck should the surgeon operate on? Would physical therapy for the neck or the shoulder be most helpful?

What if the patient with groin pain had an MRI of the groin and lumbar spine, and the MRI of the groin showed degeneration of the hip and the MRI of the lumbar spine showed a disc herniation at L4-L5 and L3-L4? Which should the doctor treat? Which should the surgeon operate on? Should physical therapy be prescribed for the hip? For the lumbar spine?

I am going to give one last example because it is one of the most common areas where patients complain of pain—the side of the hip. Is it bursitis of the hip or the lumbar spine creating the problem? What if the MRI of the hip and the spine shows degeneration in both? Does the physician put steroids into the bursa? Treat the bursa with therapy? Or treat the spine? Should the surgeon operate on the hip or the spine?

As you read the chapters in Part II that deal with your specific area of pain, I will explain how you can start to come up with a diagnosis *before* you obtain an MRI. Then you can use the MRI and the minimally invasive procedures that I will later describe to confirm the diagnosis. And answer all these questions!

I will talk more in Part III about the minimally invasive procedures that I use to help diagnose and treat the different structures in the spine that create pain, but one question that patients always ask is how they can get long-term relief from a minimally invasive procedure even though it does not fix the herniated disc or arthritic joint.

> **Remember: The inflammation around the disc herniation or arthritic joint creates the pain—not the disc herniation or arthritic joint by itself.**

I emphasize inflammation because if you eliminate the inflammation, you can live with the herniation and arthritis with minimal pain. I told you earlier that usually the body eliminates the inflammation and pain on its own. If not, all the minimally invasive procedure does is help with eradicating the inflammation by treating the irritated disc, nerve, or joint with an anti-inflammatory medication. The real trick to achieving long-term relief with this approach is not just eliminating the inflammation. That is the easy part. The difficult part is trying to keep all my patients from doing things that are going to re-aggravate their initial problem that was creating their pain, and subsequently create inflammation again! Later in the book, I will discuss body positions and exercises to keep you from re-inflaming your spine.

I am absolutely not telling you that you will never need surgery. At times, the disc, joint, or nerve is going to have recurring inflammation no matter what you do. Or the disc or nerve will create significant numbness or weakness that does not respond to conservative care. But the good thing is that you are going to know the exact problem that is creating your pain before you get it fixed.

SUMMARY

1. If you can draw on a pain diagram the area where you usually feel your pain and compare that to pictures of the human body showing the areas where the different structures of the human spine create pain, you can then start to come close to at least getting an idea of what part of the spine may be creating your pain.

2. If you can combine your pain diagram with specific information about your pain, you will be able to narrow down what may be creating your discomfort.

3. You have to locate the exact cause of your pain to be able to treat the problem.

4. You cannot always rely on an MRI to make a diagnosis, as many patients have a disc herniation and arthritis, and most will not have significant pain.

5. It is not the disc herniation or arthritis that usually creates the pain, but the inflammation around the disc or other structures of the spine.

6. You can use an MRI along with minimally invasive procedures to confirm what you already know from your pain diagram, history, and physical findings.

7. You may get long-term relief by using minimally invasive procedures and then learning how to use proper body mechanics and exercise in a way that minimizes the chance of re-inflaming the structure in your spine that was creating your pain.

8. If you fail to get long-term relief, you can use the information that shows the exact cause of your pain to help determine the type of surgery that you would need.

CHAPTER 2

Understanding the Parts of the Spine That Create Pain

THE KEY TO DIAGNOSIS

In this chapter you will not only obtain a better understanding of what part of the spine could possibly be creating your pain, but also learn how good posture and proper body movements can keep you from having discomfort.

The spine is made up of twenty-four movable bones called vertebrae that start from the bottom of your skull and end with your tailbone (**Picture 7**). The first seven bones of the neck are termed the cervical spine. The next segment, the mid-back area, is called the thoracic area and consists of twelve bones. Then comes your lower back with five bones, referred to as the lumbar spine. The bottom of the lumbar spine is connected to a large triangular bone that is called the sacrum and is wedged between the two pelvic bones. The end of the sacrum is attached to a small bone called the coccyx, which is your tailbone.

Each one of the twenty-four vertebrae is cushioned by a shock-absorbing disc, which is labeled by the bones above and below it. The letter is usually used instead of the whole word when you label the disc. For example, the disc between the fourth and fifth lumbar vertebrae is commonly labeled the L4-L5 disc. **Picture 8** shows the L4-L5 disc between the L4 and L5 vertebrae. It also shows the disc between the L5 vertebra and the sacrum. It is commonly referred to as the L5-S1 disc. This same numbering system holds true in the cervical and thoracic areas of the spine. The disc between the C6 and C7 vertebrae would be called the C6-C7 disc. The disc between the seventh thoracic vertebra and the eighth thoracic vertebra is labeled the T7-T8 disc.

In Picture 8, which shows one portion of the lumbar spine, I want to point out that the *front* of the spine contains the disc, with a vertebra on either side of it, like a hamburger in a bun. Each two vertebra are connected in the *back* of the spine by a joint, which is called a facet.

The bones and discs protect the spinal cord and nerves that are inside this structure. The spinal nerves exit through a hole between each pair of vertebrae called a foramen. You should notice in **Picture 9** that the nerve passes right by the disc, and therefore it can become irritated if the disc presses against it. Picture 9 on the bottom also includes a cross-section of

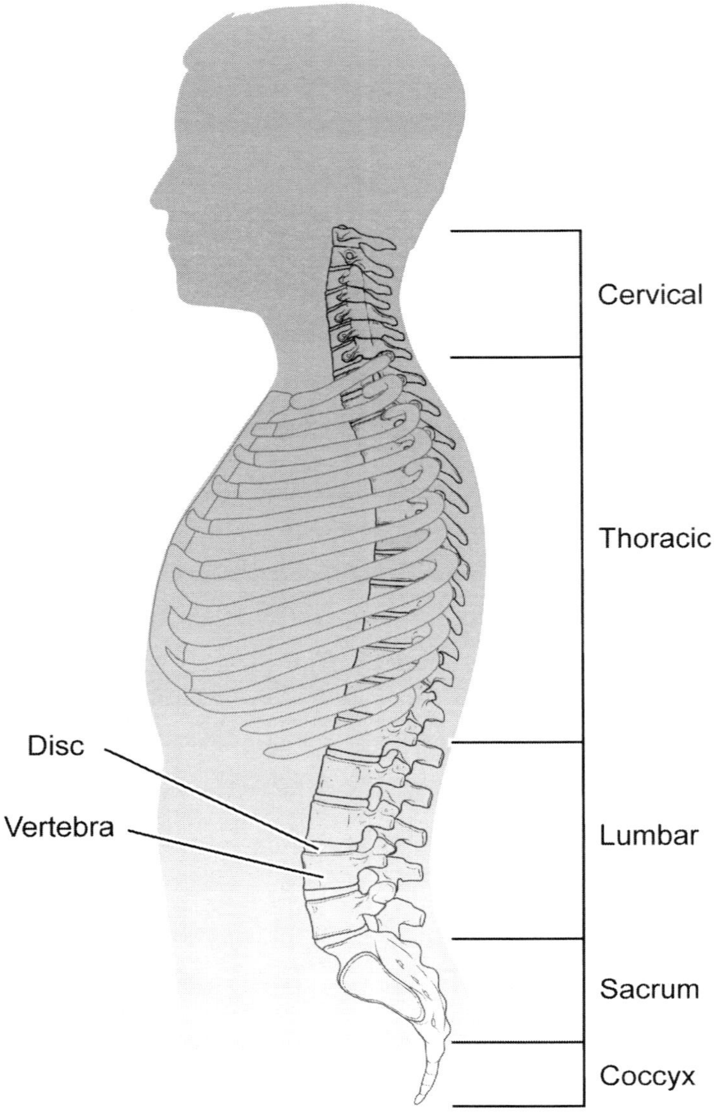

Disc

Vertebra

Cervical

Thoracic

Lumbar

Sacrum

Coccyx

The vertebrae of
the spine.

the spine, showing that the discs and facets surround the spinal canal. This
canal, when narrowed due to either a herniated disc or enlarged facets, can
become inflamed, a condition that, in turn, will irritate all the nerves running through the canal.

Three primary structures create most of the pain in the spine:

1. The disc can create pain either because the *outside* of the herniated disc
    inflames the nerve that passes by the disc, or because the *inside* of the
    disc tears and becomes inflamed.

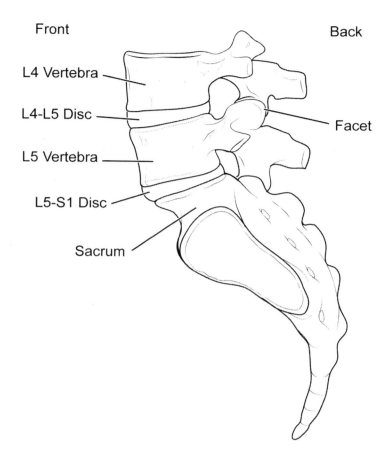

Front

Back

L4 Vertebra

L4-L5 Disc

L5 Vertebra

L5-S1 Disc

Sacrum

Facet

PICTURE 8

The front and back of the bottom part of the spine.

2. The facets—the joints between the bones in your spine—can create pain due to inflammation inside the joint, just like your knee or hip joint.

3. The nerve, which exits the hole, or foramen, on the *side* of the spine, also can create pain, either because the disc irritates the nerve as it passes by the disc, or because the hole where the nerve exits is narrowed **(Picture 10)**. The narrowing is called foraminal stenosis.

One other problem usually occurs because of a combination of these three structures. The nerves that run inside the *center* of the spinal canal can become inflamed because of the narrowing of the canal, due to either a disc herniation or enlargement of the facet joints. When the facets become enlarged because of arthritis or the disc herniates, the spinal canal will narrow and create a condition called spinal stenosis **(Picture 11)**.

Most spine pain originates from one of these four sources, and our job is to locate the specific problem that is creating the pain. As I will explain later in this chapter, it is important to know where your pain is coming from because the treatment for each one of these problems, as well as the therapy and exercises, is different.

First I want to answer a common question that I am asked all the time: can the muscles create pain? Muscles can create pain, but if it is coming from the spine, the pain usually is the result of one of the three structures—the disc, the joint, or the nerve. When one of these three structures is inflamed, the structure will send a signal through a nerve to a specific group of muscles, which in turn will create muscle spasm.

The muscle spasm coming from one of the structures of the spine is usually a *secondary issue* that will resolve itself after the inflammation in whichever structure in the spine that was creating your pain is gone. This is

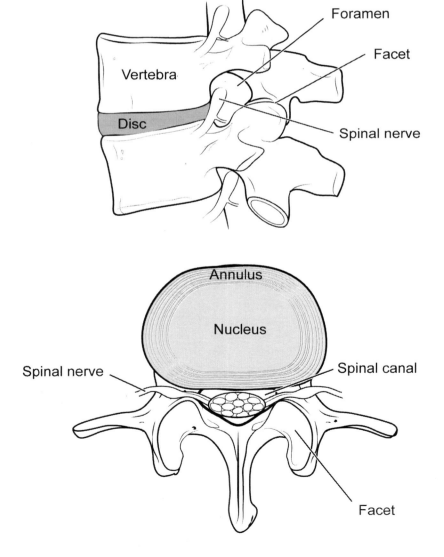

Segment of spine also showing the cross-section of the spine.

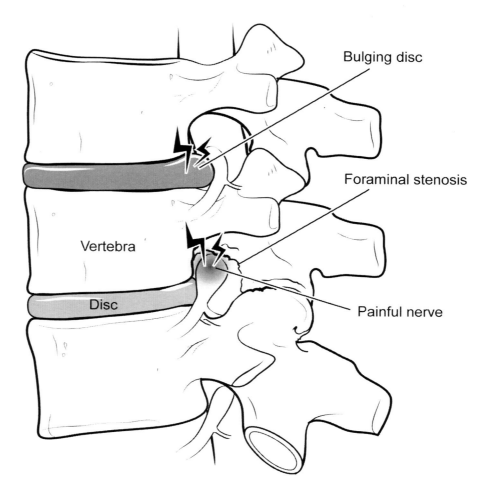

Bulging disc

Foraminal stenosis

Vertebra

Disc

Painful nerve

PICTURE 10

A bulging disc or foraminal stenosis can inflame a nerve.

going to be either a disc, joint, or nerve (or some combination of the three). During the first four to six weeks, you can treat the muscle spasm with an oral muscle relaxer as you wait for the spine pain to resolve. As I have mentioned, most spine pain will go away on its own if you just wait it out. If the muscle spasm and pain continue after the initial four to six weeks, you need to start to look for the specific cause of the muscle spasm and pain, which usually are due to one of the three structures in the spine. Treating the muscle spasm with steroid injections directly into the muscles or using a technique called "needling," in which a needle is inserted directly into the muscle with the hope of breaking up the muscle spasm, is common when we cannot identify what is creating the muscle spasms. This can be done during the first four to six weeks to help you deal with the pain; however, we now know that the muscle spasm that occurs usually is due to inflammation in one of the structures of the spine. Therefore, the better option is to treat the specific structure that is creating the pain and the muscle spasm—*not* injecting the muscles with steroids or a dry needle.

Now let's look specifically at each of these three structures that create pain. I will explain how you can almost self-diagnose the problem by learning how the structures in the spine move.

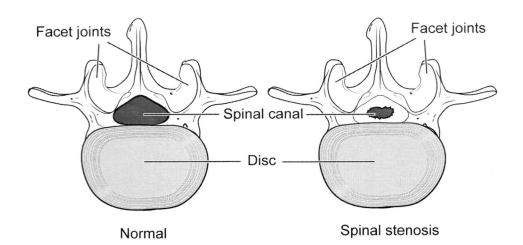

PICTURE 11

Spinal stenosis.

DISCS

Degeneration of the spinal discs is a normal aging process that occurs in everyone. The disc, like a tire, will balloon out, and the inside of the disc may even tear as we age, but in most instances, this will not create pain. A lot of patients are told they have degenerated discs and are given the feeling that they have some sort of disease. *We all are going to have degenerated discs!* Some of us may have changes in our discs earlier than others because of genetics or because of escapades in our youth, but no one is going to escape the gradual drying out and bulging of the discs (**Picture 12**).

Half the world population has some form of degenerative or herniated disc disease by the time they are in their fifties, and they will have absolutely *no* pain. Most disc herniations are going to create pain only if the disc becomes inflamed, or if the disc inflames the nerve. I keep repeating this because this concept is essential. I have patients who are under the impression that all herniated discs seen on their MRI have to be creating pain and, in turn, need to be treated or operated on to give them long-term relief. However, in most cases, your body is going to eliminate the inflammation in the first four to six weeks. If you then change the way you move, and exercise so that you can use other parts of your body and not your spine for your daily activities, you can usually live pain-free without treating or cutting on the discs.

> **Remember: Discs do not create pain unless they become inflamed. You can live with herniated discs all your life and have minimal pain unless they become inflamed.**

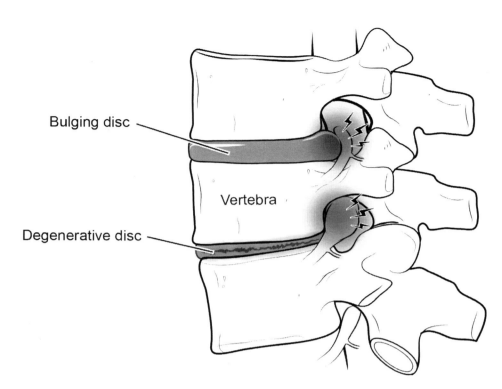

Bulging disc

Vertebra

Degenerative disc

Bulging and
degenerative discs.

The terminology used for degenerated discs can vary. "Herniated," "protruding," and "bulging" are all terms that are used to describe this condition. One of the most common questions that I am asked is what the difference is between a herniated, protruding, or bulging disc. This terminology may be used to categorize discs by size, with a protruding or bulging disc being smaller in size and the herniated disc being the larger disc. But none of this matters. What does matter is whether the disc creates pain, numbness, or weakness—and if it does create one of these three problems, it may have nothing to do with the size or shape of the disc. I have treated patients with huge herniated discs with minimal pain and others who have small bulging discs with significant pain.

When a disc becomes inflamed, it will create pain. The pain that comes from these discs can be due to either the outside of the disc irritating a nerve, or the inside of the disc, called the annulus, tearing and becoming inflamed.

When the disc protrudes or herniates, and the *outside* of the disc inflames the nerve, as seen in the top image of **Picture 13**, the pain can go all the way down the arm or leg, or wrap around your ribs, or may just create back, mid-back, or neck pain, depending on which nerve is affected. If the *inside* of the disc is inflamed because of a tear in the border of the disc, called the annulus, as seen in the bottom image of Picture 13, the pain usually will not go down the arm or leg but instead affect the central area of the body, meaning the neck, mid-back, or lower back, depending on which disc is inflamed.

Let's talk about the mechanics of the discs. Once you know how they move, you will get a better understanding of what inflames the discs and what you can do to prevent them from becoming irritated.

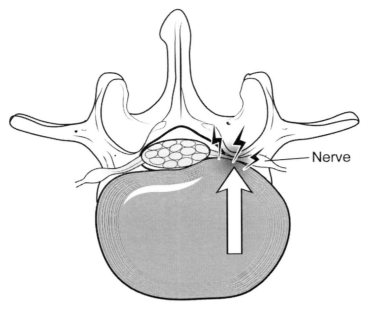

Nerve

Disc herniation

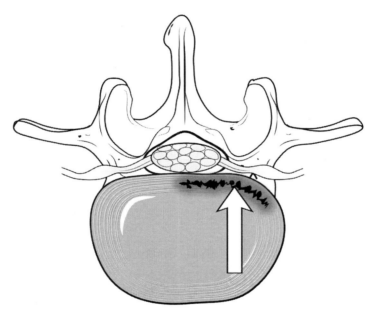

Annular tear

PICTURE 13

Two discs: (top) the outside of the disc herniation pressing on a nerve, creating inflammation, and (bottom) the inside of the disc with tears and inflammation.

In **Picture 14**, note that the discs are located in the front of the spine, acting as a cushion between the vertebrae.

Therefore, if you bend forward from the waist without bending your knees when you pick things up off the floor, reach for things on a low shelf, or brush your teeth, the pressure on the disc increases. This increase in pressure over a period of time can inflame the disc or irritate the nerve. The human spine was not meant to bend from the waist. *We were made to bend our knees and keep the back straight.* In the long term, you will have less pain if you can do your daily activities by bending your knees instead of your back because you will keep the disc from becoming inflamed (**Picture 15**).

A comment I hear repeatedly from patients is that, for whatever reason, they cannot bend their knees, and therefore they feel that they have to bend their backs. In that case, you should sit or use a stool when you do those activities that usually require bending of the knees, such as emptying the dishwasher or taking clothes out of the washing machine, as that will put less pressure on the discs. Or use some of the tools that have a grabber on one end that lets you pick up things without bending.

The increased pressure that comes from bending and twisting activities may create inflammation inside the disc, which will result in back pain. The other problem that can occur from repeated bending of the lower back instead of the legs is that the disc can irritate the lumbar nerves and cause them to become inflamed. In this situation, you may feel pain going down the legs. Most patients with disc pain hurt worse when they are in a sitting position as that increases the pressure inside the disc. People with disc pain also may notice significant pain when moving from a sitting to standing position, particularly if they have been sitting for a long time at a desk or in a car. An activity that helps patients with disc pain is walking, because that does not allow body weight and gravity to pressurize the disc.

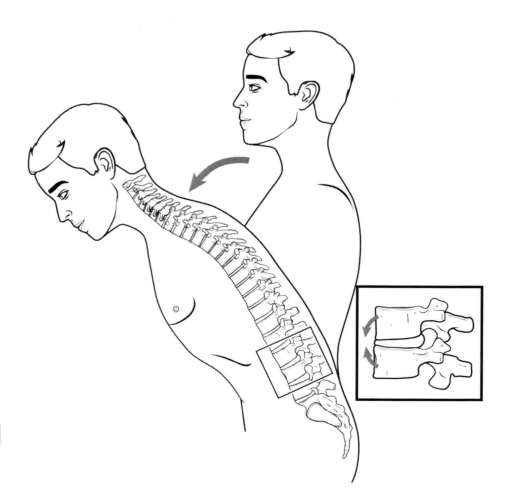

PICTURE 14

Bending forward puts pressure on the disc.

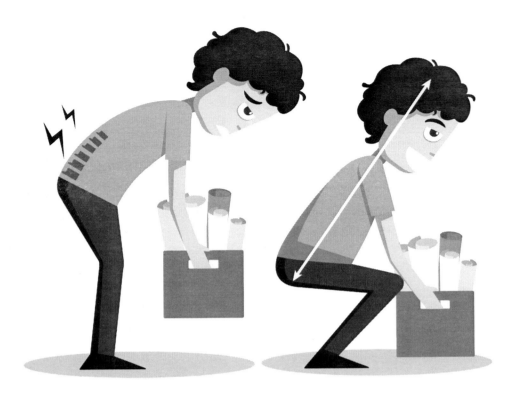

PICTURE 15

Proper posture when you pick something up involves bending the knees.

As mentioned, sitting for long periods of time can create increased pressure on the discs. Whether you have pain or not, as the years go by and you keep sitting for long periods of time, you are going to increase the possibility of finally inflaming the discs. Therefore, I tell patients not to stay in one position for long periods of time, as just getting up for a few minutes every hour or so will take pressure off the discs and reduce the possibility of inflammation. If you do have a job that requires a lot of sitting, I recommend that you get a desk that allows you to both sit and stand. You can change positions every thirty minutes or so, which will decrease the possibility of inflaming the discs. Make sure you also keep your back straight when you do have to sit, as slumping forward will create the same problem as bending your back when you lift something, which is to place a lot of pressure on your discs.

This same concept about bending your spine applies to the neck. The discs in the neck are called the cervical discs and are in the *front* of your spine, right behind your windpipe (trachea) **(Picture 16)**. When you bend your head forward to look down to do something, like reading, sewing, or even just using your phone, you place a lot of pressure on these discs.

If your cervical disc is inflamed, you may notice that your neck may hurt when you are looking down for an extended period of time. A lot more pressure is placed on these discs when your head is bent forward. Cervical discs can create pain in the neck and shoulders, or if the disc irritates the nerves, you may notice pain going down the arms. Positions like sitting in front of a

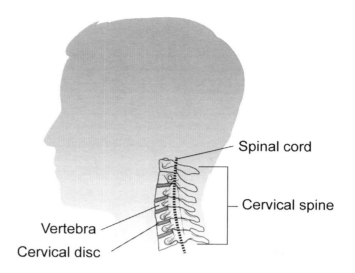

Spinal cord

Cervical spine

Vertebra

Cervical disc

computer or looking down at your laptop will increase the chance of inflaming the cervical discs and nerves.

The same points that I have made for the lumbar and cervical spine also hold true for the mid-back (otherwise called the thoracic spine). Repeated bending at the mid-back level or sitting in a slumped position can aggravate the discs in the thoracic spine, which will create pain in the mid-back **(Picture 17)**, which is the area from the top of the shoulder blades all the way down into the upper back. If the disc irritates the nerve, you may feel the pain wrapping around your ribs.

> **Remember: Do not bend forward from the low back, mid-back, or neck for long periods of time, as this places a lot of pressure on your discs. Do not sit for long periods of time, as doing so will create increased pressure on the discs and possibly inflame them.**

If you have pain coming from your discs, you may find yourself arching backward at times so that you take the pressure off the inflamed disc. Or you may notice yourself trying to hold yourself up with your arms when you are sitting down to reduce pressure on the disc. This is a type of auto- or self-traction. Patients with disc pain also usually feel better in the morning because no gravity or body weight is being placed on the discs while you're lying down. For these people, the pain gets worse throughout the day after prolonged sitting or twisting activities.

Chapter 17 will review this concept in detail as I teach you proper body mechanics to avoid painful periods with your spine, whether it is your neck, mid-back, or lower back.

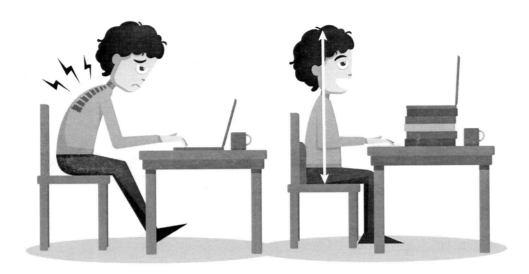

Proper posture when you sit at a computer.

DISC PAIN

1. The discs are in the front of your spine and can create pain either in your neck, mid-back, or lower back depending on which disc you inflame. If the cervical discs are inflamed, they will create pain in the neck and shoulders; if it is one of the thoracic discs, it will create pain in the middle of your back; and if it is a lumbar disc that is irritated, you will experience lower back and buttock pain. Because there are nerves inside the disc, you may have disc pain even without having a herniation.

2. If the nerve next to the disc becomes inflamed as a result of the disc irritating the nerve, you may experience pain in any area where the nerve travels in the body.

3. Certain positions will aggravate the discs and the nerves. Bending the spine forward and twisting are two movements you should reduce to keep your discs from becoming inflamed. For example, you create increased pressure on the disc in your cervical spine when you look down while working at your computer or reading, the thoracic disc is at risk for becoming irritated if you are slumped over your desk at work, and your lumbar discs are being overworked when you pick up things without bending your knees.

4. Learn to keep your spine straight no matter what you do and use your arms and legs to help you lift things. Squat and bend your knees as much as possible to keep the pressure off your discs.

5. Do not stay in one position for long periods of time. Try to stand up from a sitting position every thirty minutes and learn to stretch by arching your back to take the pressure off your discs.

6. If you do have pain coming from the disc, you may notice that you will tend *not* to want to sit for long periods of time and you may tend to arch your spine to give yourself relief, as that gives the disc more breathing room. You also may notice yourself sitting with your hands pressing down against the chair as you try to support your back. This is actually a form of auto-traction as you try to take the pressure off the discs.

JOINTS OR FACETS

The joints commonly are called facets and are located in the *back* of the spine **(Picture 18)**.

The facet joints join the vertebrae together in the back of the spine and they have cartilage that wraps around the joint and provides cushion for the joint. Each joint is named by a combination of the vertebrae above and below it. Therefore, the L4-L5 joint or facet is the joint between the fourth and fifth lumbar vertebrae. These joints run from the bottom of the skull all

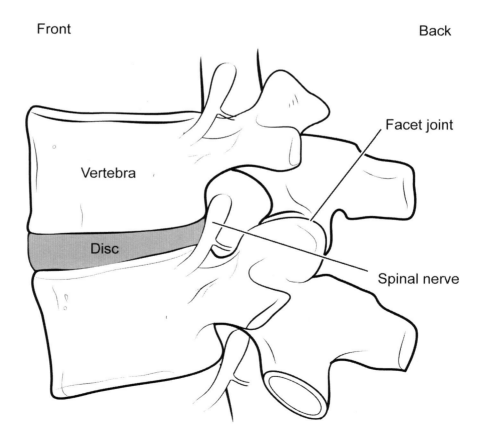

Front   Back

Facet joint

Vertebra

Disc

Spinal nerve

PICTURE 18

Facet joint.

the way down to the last lumbar vertebra. So, for example, the joint between the sixth and seventh cervical vertebrae is the C6-C7 joint or facet.

The joints move in the exact opposite direction of the discs. They open up when your spine bends forward, which is called flexion, and they close on top of each other when you bend backward, which is called extension. When your joints become inflamed and painful, you will notice that as you arch or bend your spine backward, the pain becomes worse, whereas if you slump forward or bend your head down, you usually experience less pain. This is exactly the opposite of disc pain, which gets worse when your spine bends forward (**Picture 19**).

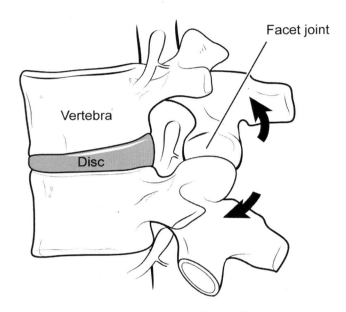

Flexion (bending forward)

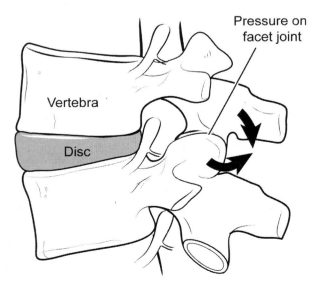

Extension
(arching the back or bending backward)

PICTURE 19

Facet joints open when you bend forward and press on each other when you bend backward.

Just like the discs, when facets become arthritic or degenerated, they will usually *not* become painful until they become inflamed. So, just because an MRI shows arthritis in the joints in your spine, this does not mean they will create pain. Patients tell me that they have been diagnosed with arthritis and therefore they have pain. Most facets or joints create no pain, no matter how arthritic they are.

The joints in the human spine create axial pain, which means that the pain is in the neck and back areas without going down the arms or legs. **Picture 20** shows where you would feel pain depending on which facet joint is inflamed. The image on the left shows the cervical facets and the image on the right shows the lumbar facets. For example, if you look at the image on the left, you will see that when the C5-C6 facet is inflamed, the pain will be in the lower neck and the back of the shoulder. If the C2-C3 facet is inflamed, the pain will be in the top of the neck and the skull. If you look at the image on the right, you can see that when the L5-S1 facet is inflamed it will create pain in the lower back going down into the buttock. The L3-L4 facet when inflamed will cause pain only in the back.

> **Remember: Facet pain will never create pain going down the arms or legs.**

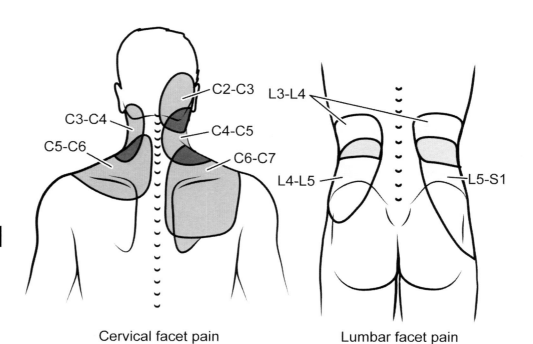

PICTURE 20

Different areas of the body where you will feel pain depending on which facet is inflamed.

Cervical facet pain   Lumbar facet pain

Joint pain is usually worse when you arch backward, whether it is your neck or back, and gets better when you lean forward. This is exactly the opposite of disc pain.

> **Remember: The discs are in the front of your spine and the joints are in the back. Therefore, when you bend forward you press on the discs and when you bend backward you press on the joints.**

Most people with joint pain slump forward when they are sitting, because it hurts to sit up straight. When people with facet pain sleep, they do not like to lie on their backs because as the spine straightens, the joints are going to press on each other, and if the joints are inflamed, they will create pain. If your pain is coming from the joints, you may notice yourself tossing or turning at night, or you may awaken in the morning with significant pain from the joints pressing on each other all night. You may feel better if you sleep on your side in a fetal position so that you can keep your joints open at night. Throughout the day, the discomfort from inflamed joints gets better as you usually sit or walk with a little slump, which opens up the joints. Standing in one position also creates pain, as the joints will press on each other, but as soon as you start walking, you will feel better as you tend to bend forward a little bit when you walk.

The same thing holds true with the neck. When you have pain coming from the joints in the neck, you may notice that it will usually hurt when you look up and feel better when you are looking down. Neck pain due to facet inflammation also creates more pain at night.

FACET PAIN

1. If you have pain coming from the facets or joints in the lower back, it usually feels worse when you arch or twist your back, and it gets better when you bend forward. You will notice the pain more when you sit up straight because the inflamed joints will press on each other, and you will feel better when you slump forward.

2. You also may notice that trying to get up from a sitting position is painful, as the facet joints will press on each other as you go through that motion.

3. Standing in one place may increase your pain as your spine is in a straight or slightly arched position, but you will usually feel better once you start to walk.

4. If the joints in your neck are involved, you may notice that you experience more pain when you arch your head backward, and you feel better when you look down.

5. You also may notice that sleeping is difficult, because when you lie down and straighten your back, the joints press on each other. Therefore, you may feel better when you sleep on your side.

6. The first few minutes after getting out of bed can be really rough because the inflamed facets have been pressing on each other while you were lying down, but after you get moving, the pain will be reduced.

NERVES

The nerves are the only parts of the spine that create pain that goes down the arms and legs. **Picture 21** shows the path of all the nerves in the spine and the different areas that they cover on the *surface* of the body. The nerves in the neck are called the cervical nerves, the ones in the mid-back the thoracic nerves, and the ones in the lower back area the lumbar nerves. When one of the nerves is inflamed, it will create pain in the area of the body shown in the picture. For example, if the sixth cervical nerve, labeled C6 in Picture 21, is inflamed, you may notice pain starting in the neck and shoulder or the arm going down to your thumb and first finger. If the tenth thoracic nerve, T10 in Picture 21, is inflamed, you may have pain starting in the mid-back wrapping around to the front of your abdomen. If the fourth lumbar nerve, L4 in Picture 21, is inflamed, you can have pain anywhere from the back and buttock area all the way down to the foot.

The nerves exit through a hole formed by the bones. The medical term for this hole is a foramen, through which the nerves descend in their respective paths down the body. For example, in **Picture 22**, the fourth lumbar nerve (L4) comes out between the fourth and fifth lumbar vertebrae through the foramen. Picture 22 shows that a disc herniation may inflame the nerve that passes by the disc.

Each nerve root consists of a bundle of different types of nerves that are wrapped together. The three most important types are motor nerves (which can create weakness when inflamed), sensory nerves (which create numbness when inflamed), and pain fibers. Patients ask questions about this important concept all the time. They want to know why sometimes they

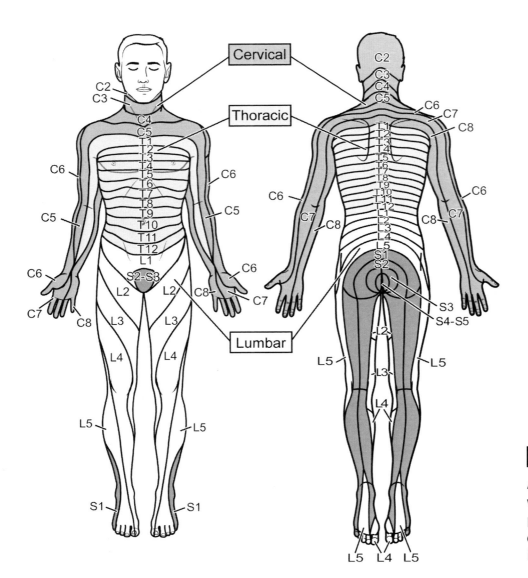

Areas of the body where you will feel pain depending on which nerve is inflamed.

have pain going down their arms or legs and other times they feel numbness or weakness. You may notice different symptoms depending on which part of the nerve is affected, even though it is the *same* nerve. For example, you may notice that your shoulder hurts, your bicep is weak, and your thumb is numb; all three of these symptoms are due to the C6 nerve. Or, if the L4 nerve is inflamed, you may have buttock pain and tingling and numbness in the foot.

Remember one other very important thing about nerve pain: it usually will come and go, affecting different areas along the path of the nerve at different times. One time, the C6 nerve may create pain in the back of the shoulder; another time, you may notice pain and tingling in the arm; the next time, all you notice is numbness in the thumb. Or you have some combination of these symptoms, like shoulder pain with numbness in the fingers, but no arm pain. Another example of this pain variation would be

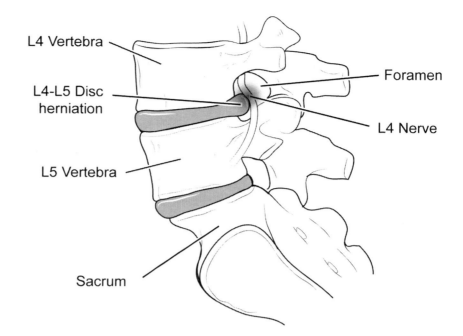

PICTURE 22

L4 nerve inflamed by the L4-L5 disc herniation.

the L4 nerve creating buttock pain with numbness in your foot one time and pain in your shin the next time.

Patients with nerve pain also can have swelling in their hands and feet depending on whether the inflamed nerve is in the neck or the back. You can have swelling in the hands when the nerve in the neck is inflamed and swelling of the legs and feet if the nerve in the back is inflamed.

Earlier in this chapter, I explained that nerves in the lumbar spine can become inflamed in two different places—the *side* of the spine where the nerve exits or the *center* of the canal of the spine. It is important to determine which one of the two is creating your pain because the treatment, therapy, and exercises for each one of these problems are quite different.

Lumbar Side Nerve Pain

The leg pain, numbness, and/or weakness in lumbar *side* nerve pain is caused by a disc herniation in the spine creating inflammation of the nerve or by arthritis narrowing the hole where the nerve exits, causing the nerve to become inflamed. **Picture 23** shows a bulging disc pushing on the nerve as well as another nerve being inflamed because of an arthritic narrowed hole, which is called foraminal stenosis.

Picture 21 shows the common standard "dermatome chart" depicting where every nerve in the spine covers the *surface* of the human body. If a lumbar nerve is inflamed, the pain will be in the areas shown in **Picture 24**.

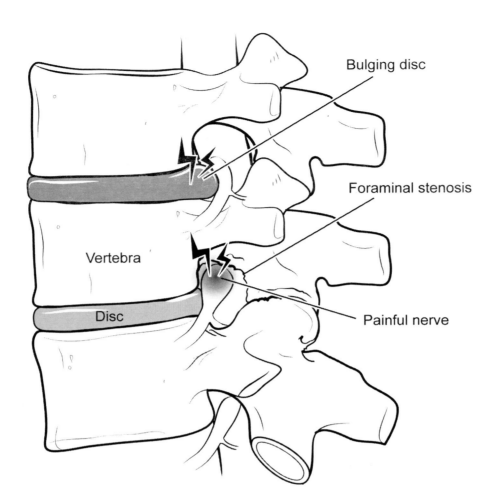

Bulging disc

Foraminal stenosis

Vertebra

Disc

Painful nerve

Bulging disc or foraminal stenosis can inflame a nerve.

So if the L5 nerve is inflamed, you can have pain, numbness, or weakness starting in the back and buttock area and going down the side of the leg to the foot. If the L3 nerve is irritated, you may notice that pain, numbness, or weakness starts in the back and wraps around to the front of the leg. One thing to keep in mind is that Picture 24 shows only the skin area where you will feel the symptoms. **Picture 25** shows the same nerves, but instead of showing the *surface* of the body that they cover, it shows the different *muscles* and *bones* that the nerves go to in the lower part of the body.

It is important to know that you can feel pain, numbness, or weakness in the areas shown in Picture 24, but at the same time, you may have muscle and bone pain in the areas shown in Picture 25. For example, if you look at Picture 24, you see that the L5 nerve can create pain and numbness starting in the back, wrapping around the hip, and moving down the lateral part of the leg all the way to the toes. If you look at Picture 25, you can see all the muscles and bones that the L5 nerve covers, including the groin, the area over the side of your hip, and the lower buttock. If you combine these two pictures, you can see that the L5 nerve starts in the back, goes down into the side of the hip, moves to the lower buttock and groin, and then continues down the side of the leg to

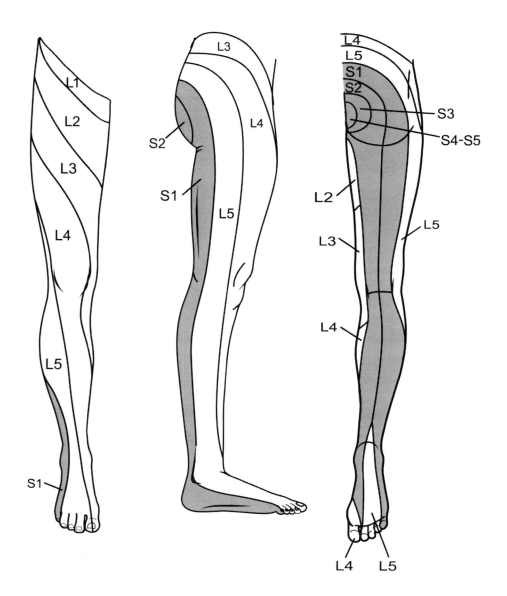

PICTURE 24

Areas of the body where you will feel pain when the lumbar nerves are inflamed.

the toes. **Picture 26** shows the combination of Pictures 24 and 25, depicting all the areas that you could feel pain if the L5 nerve is inflamed. Always look at both pictures when you are trying to decide where your pain is coming from!

Let us look at another nerve, the L4 from the lumbar spine. Following the L4 nerve in Picture 24, you will notice how it can create pain in the side of the hip, wrap around to the front of the thigh and shin, and then go down to the front of the toes. Picture 25 points out the muscles and bones that the L4 nerve goes to. When you look at Picture 25, you notice that the L4 nerve also covers the groin area, the lower buttock, and the area where the bursa of the hip is located on the side of the hip. Combine these two pictures (**Picture 27**) and you see that the L4 nerve starts in the back, wraps around the hip, goes into the groin and deep into the buttock, and finishes up in the thigh, shin, and front of the foot. Chapter 4 provides more information on *side* nerve pain coming from the lumbar spine.

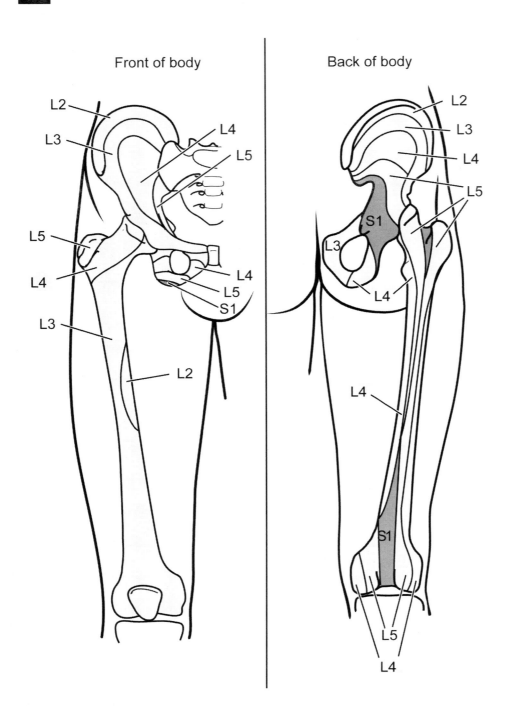

Front of body

Back of body

PICTURE 25

Nerves in the lumbar spine can create pain in the muscles and bones of the hip, buttock, and groin when inflamed.

You can have pain in one area that the nerve goes to without having any discomfort in the rest of the path of the nerve. For example, the L4 nerve may produce pain in the side of the hip, but no back or leg pain. Or that same nerve may create leg pain, but no hip or back pain. Or it produces back pain, but no hip or leg pain. And every one of these different presentations is coming from the same L4 nerve.

Why am I making such a big deal of where these nerves run? Because a lot of patients come to see me with pain on the side of their leg, lower buttock, or in their groin and have been told that their pain is coming from

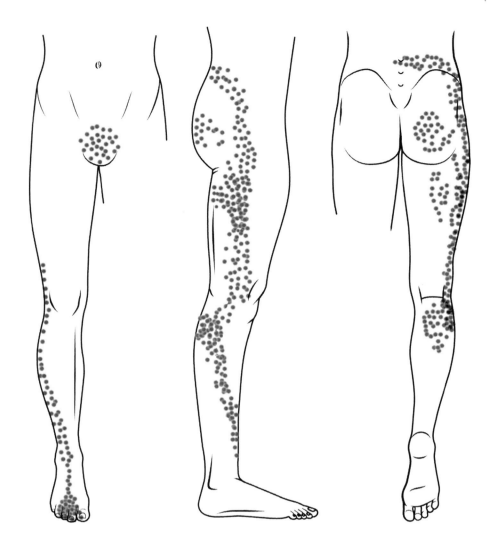

PICTURE 26

All the areas of the body that can hurt when the L5 nerve is inflamed.

the hip joint or their hip bursa, but it turns out their pain was coming from one of their lumbar nerves. I always tell patients to look at *both* Pictures 24 and 25 when they are trying to diagnose the nerve that is creating their pain because Picture 24 covers the *surface* of the body and Picture 25 covers the *muscles* and *bones*. Chapter 7 discusses hip pain in more detail.

Most patients will tell me that their nerve pain was not triggered by a specific event but started spontaneously. They may have awoken with the pain or just noticed that their back pain started with a little muscle ache and became worse over a period of days. And then a day later, the leg might have started to hurt. Spine pain, whether it originates in the disc, nerve, or joint, does not start the same way all the time, and you do not have to be doing some strenuous activity when your pain starts. The body can get rid of a certain amount of inflammation, but once it gets above a certain point, you will start to hurt. You may have started the inflammatory process a few days earlier while you were lifting something the wrong way, but you never felt any pain because the level of inflammation was not high enough. Then, after

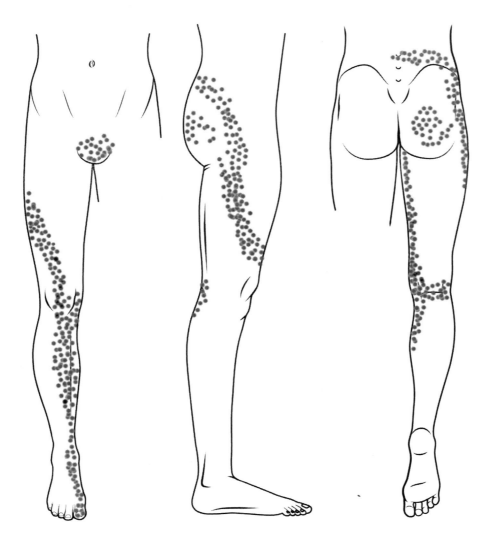

PICTURE 27

All the areas of the body that can hurt when the L4 nerve is inflamed.

doing your daily activities, which may have included sitting for a long time or taking things out of your car without bending your knees, you may have noticed a little bit of soreness, but not any significant pain. However, the amount of inflammation could still be increasing. You then go to sleep and wake up dying in pain, and you wonder why you are hurting even though all you were doing was resting. What happened is that the inflammation finally got to a point that it created pain. Your daily activities, especially if not done using proper body mechanics, may start the inflammation around the disc and the nerve even though you do not feel pain.

When it comes to the lumbar or lower back area, you will notice that sitting or driving makes the pain from the nerve worse, and when you stand up, it feels better. **Picture 28** demonstrates why that happens. The lumbar nerve is the shortest when you are in the standing position and stretches when you sit. Imagine the line that you see going down the leg to be the nerve. The sitting position pulls on the nerve as it gets bent. If the nerve is inflamed, it may create pain in that position.

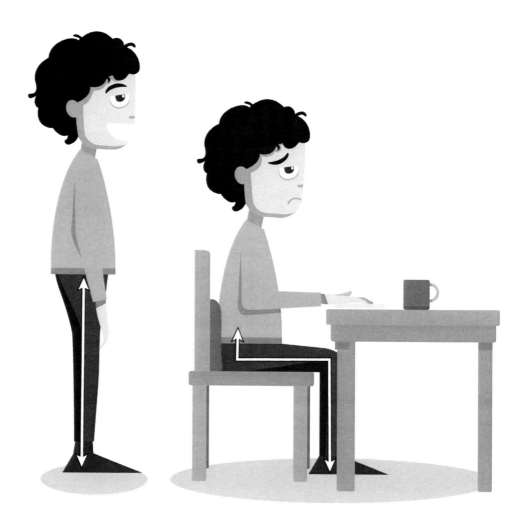

PICTURE 28

Stretching of the
nerve when you move
to a sitting position.

The other problem with sitting is that this position will put the most
pressure on the disc because of body weight and gravity. If the disc and nerve
are inflamed, this position is going to create pain. As you can see, the sitting
position for a person with a disc herniation and inflamed nerve is not good
for two reasons. The pulling of the nerve and the pressure of the disc against
the nerve in the sitting position can both create pain. Bending forward may
make the pain worse if the pain is due to a disc pressing on a nerve. Patients
tell me that even brushing their teeth can hurt when their pain is coming
from the disc and nerve.

Arching the back may help push the disc away from the nerve and give
some level of relief. Standing and walking can make the discomfort less by
not allowing the body's weight and gravity to put all their pressure on the
disc and by decreasing the stretch in the nerve, which, in turn, will minimize
the irritation of the nerve.

The sciatic nerve, which is often described as any nerve going down the
back of the leg, is actually made up of three different nerve roots coming

together to form one nerve. These three are the L4, L5, and S1 nerves. "Sciatica" is a common term for any nerve pain that you feel going down the leg, but it actually means that one of these three nerve roots is inflamed because either a disc is pressing on a nerve or the narrowing of the hole (foramen) is creating an irritation of the nerve. Nerve pain is usually worse at night, either because the position of your body aggravates the nerve or because you are not distracted by thinking about other things as you do during the day.

Lumbar Center Pain

We just discussed nerve pain in the back and leg when the disc is herniated and pressing on the nerve, or when the foramen—the hole on the *side* of the vertebra—is narrowed (Picture 23).

Another type of nerve pain in the lumbar spine occurs when the hole in the *center* of the spine becomes narrowed because of a disc herniation or because the joints in the spine become enlarged as a result of arthritis. This narrowing of the spinal canal is called spinal or central stenosis. This type of stenosis is more common in men and women over the age of fifty.

Picture 29 shows this narrowing in the *center* of the canal of the spine where all the nerves run. When the nerves become inflamed as a result of the irritation caused by the narrowed canal, you can start to have pain.

The pain from this type of stenosis always gets worse when you walk or stand in one place. It gets dramatically better when you sit down. Remember, when the nerve is inflamed because of the narrowing of the hole on the *side* of the vertebra, or because of a disc herniation pressing on the nerve as it exits the hole on the *side* of the vertebra (Picture 23), the symptoms are usually the complete opposite. Walking when you have a nerve problem on the *side* of the spine reduces the pain, while sitting aggravates it. This piece of information is

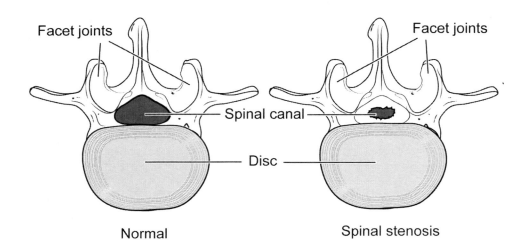

Normal   Spinal stenosis

PICTURE 29

Central spinal stenosis.

important because you and your health-care practitioner can tell exactly where the problem is located depending on what makes the pain better or worse.

In spinal stenosis the *center* canal is narrowed, and standing up straight makes the stenosis worse (**Picture 30**). When you lean forward, the central canal opens and gives the nerves more breathing room.

Therefore, people with spinal stenosis will bend forward at times in order to reduce the pain and may even walk that way. They will sleep on their side in a fetal position, as sleeping on their back will straighten the spine and create pain and stiffness in the morning. A common sign that I use when I am trying to determine whether patients have spinal stenosis is the "shopping cart" sign. Patients with spinal stenosis may walk around the supermarket bent over holding on to the grocery cart because that specific position will open their spine, give the nerves more breathing room, and therefore create less pain. These patients' family members may pester them to stand up straight, not understanding that the bent-over position eases the patients' pain. By straightening up, these patients actually create more problems by closing down their spine. I even encourage these patients to use a walker or at least a cane so they can lean on it. This bent-forward position allows the spinal canal to stay open. A walker with an attached seat is even better, because every half hour or so, the patient can sit down for several minutes, which in turn will decrease the swelling of the nerves. If you have spinal stenosis but do not use a walker, find someplace to sit down every thirty minutes for four or five minutes. Most importantly, you need to do

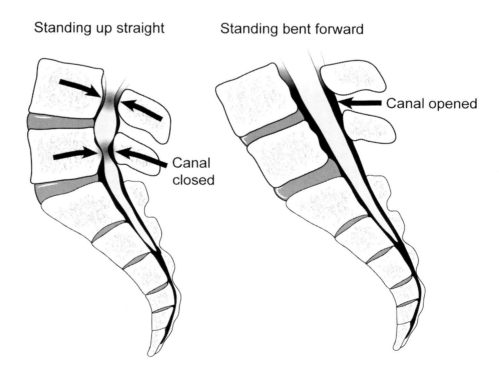

PICTURE 30

The spinal canal opens when you bend forward.

this even when you are not hurting, because sitting will decrease the chance of the nerves getting inflamed, thus reducing recurrences of pain.

You probably are wondering why I am making such a big deal of whether the problem is in the *central* area of the spine, which usually is due to stenosis and causes pain when walking (Picture 29), or whether the problem is the result of *side* stenosis, caused by the bony narrowing of the foramen or the result of a disc herniation pressing on the nerve as it exits the foramen, causing pain while sitting (Picture 23). Diagnosis is essential because all the treatments, physical therapy, exercises, and preventive body positions are exactly the opposite depending on the problem.

The following box summarizes the differences between *central* and *side* nerve pain:

THE DIFFERENCE BETWEEN SIDE LUMBAR NERVE PAIN AND CENTRAL NERVE PAIN

Side Nerve Pain

Side nerve pain occurs when the disc is pushing on the nerve as it exits the foramen or when the foramen is narrowed due to arthritic changes. Patients complain of the following:

1. Pain is worse when you sit and gets better when you walk.

2. The pain is usually on one side.

3. The pain typically gets worse when you bend forward and usually feels better when you arch the back. If the disc herniation is large enough, it can create *both* side and central nerve pain. In that situation, bending forward may actually feel better.

4. Side nerve pain may feel better during the day if you do not sit a lot, and then become worse at night. This may be due to the position you sleep in, or just because there are fewer distractions, and therefore your brain becomes more concentrated on the nerve pain.

5. Side nerve pain that is caused by arthritis narrowing the foramen, or due to a disc herniation, can occur in the lumbar, thoracic, and cervical spine.

Central Nerve Pain

Central nerve pain occurs when a disc herniation or arthritis creates narrowing of the center of the spinal canal (otherwise known as central spinal stenosis). Patients complain of the following:

1. The pain is worse when you stand or walk and gets better when you sit.

2. The pain can be on both sides of the back and involve both legs.

3. The pain is worse when you stand up straight and gets better when you bend forward.

4. The pain is worse at night and you may notice cramps in the legs.

5. Getting out of bed may be difficult, as your back may feel stiff and ache.

6. Central nerve pain usually occurs in the lumbar spine.

You have one more thing to remember: you can have *both* side nerve pain and central nerve pain at the same time if the disc or the stenosis is creating the problem on the side *and* in the center of the spine. In that situation, you may notice that it is hard to sit or stand for long periods of time.

Chapter 4 addresses side nerve pain and Chapter 6 addresses central nerve pain. Here I want to mention two last symptoms of nerve inflammation: swelling of the hands and feet and muscle spasms.

Swelling of the Hands and Feet

When the nerves of the cervical or lumbar spine are inflamed or compressed, you may notice swelling in the hands and feet. This swelling is due to a specific part of the nerve, called the sympathetic system, becoming activated as a result of the inflammation or compression of the nerves. You may have a few other symptoms other than the swelling, or you may notice that you have arm and leg pain with the swelling. Just remember, if you have swelling in one or both legs and feet and you have a history of back pain, the two may have something to do with each other. If you have ruled out other causes, you should consider that the swelling of your legs and feet may be caused by a problem with your lumbar spine. In the same fashion, if you have arm pain and notice that your hand is swollen, it could be due to the inflammation of the nerves in the neck. Once the inflammation of the nerve subsides, either spontaneously or with treatment, the swelling in the extremities will go away.

Muscle Spasms

Let's talk about muscle spasms one more time. All the structures of the spine that we have discussed so far—discs, nerves, and joints—create spasms in the muscles along the spine when the structure is inflamed. The muscle spasm is due to a nerve from the structure sending signals to the muscle telling the muscle that the structure is irritated, and subsequently the muscle spasm occurs to stabilize the inflamed structure. It is okay to treat muscle spasms with muscle relaxants and physical therapy during the first four to six weeks because most of the inflammation of the spine is going to be gone after that period. *But*, if the muscle spasm continues past that time period, it is time to look for the culprit that is *creating* the muscle spasm instead of just *treating* the muscle spasm pain. Muscle spasms will not resolve in the long term until the inflamed structure heals, either spontaneously or with treatment. Instead of having trigger point injections with dry needling, steroids, or Botox injected into the muscles, you would be better off treating the structure that is creating the problem and not the muscle. Once the inflammation in the structure is gone, the muscle spasms will stop.

Cervical Nerve Pain

When the nerve is inflamed in the neck, it can create pain that radiates into the arm, shoulder, or neck. The pain can be either in the front of the shoulder or the back of it. **Picture 31** shows the locations where each nerve in the cervical spine creates pain. Some of the nerves not only go down the arm but also create pain in the back or front of the shoulders and even up the neck all the way to the skull. Remember, the pain from the nerves can also go to the muscles of the neck and the shoulder. To get the full picture of where the nerve creates pain, you should combine the areas inside the box with the images outside the box.

You may not feel the pain along the whole length of the nerve *all* the time. You may have only neck, shoulder, or arm pain (or a combination of those three) even though the pain is coming from the same nerve. Remember that the dysfunction of the nerve can create a combination of pain, numbness, and weakness. So you may notice that you have pain in the back of the shoulder blade, weakness in the arm, and numbness in the fingers. Or you may experience just numbness in the fingers and nothing else. Or you may have pain in the shoulder blade and nothing else. You do not have to have neck pain even though the nerve that is creating your problem starts in the neck. **Picture 32** shows a typical patient with pain from the C7 nerve. As you can see, there is pain going down the arm as well as into the shoulder blade.

The neck or arm pain at times may increase when you bend your neck either up or down, and the pain from an inflamed nerve in the cervical spine usually gets worse when you turn your head to the same side that your pain is on. Patients with neck and arm pain may turn their head to the side opposite of their pain to give the nerve more room. You may even notice that holding your arm over your head relieves the pain, as that position will relax the nerve by lifting it away from the disc. Chapters 8, 9, and 10 go into more detail about neck and arm pain.

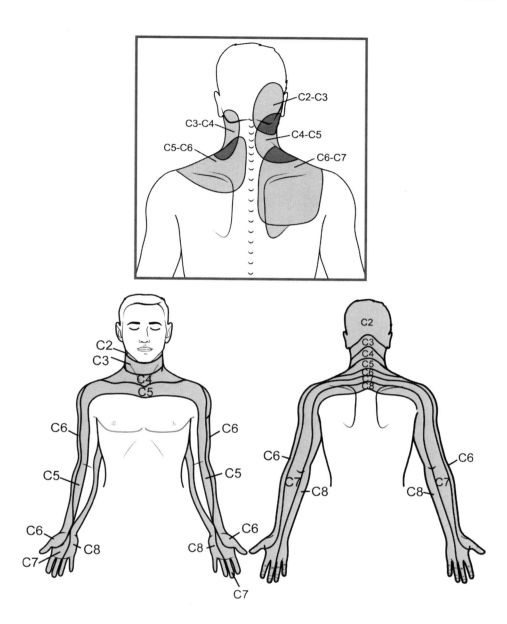

PICTURE 31

Areas of the body that will be painful when specific cervical nerves are inflamed.

Thoracic Nerve Pain

Nerve pain in the thoracic or mid-back area is actually a lot more common than people think. **Picture 33** shows the area of the body that the thoracic nerves cover. The thoracic nerves start at the bottom of the neck and go all the way down to the upper back.

If you look at Picture 33, you will notice that each nerve of the thoracic spine starts from the back of the spine and goes all the way around to the front of the body.

Each nerve is attached to the bottom of the rib and follows the path of the rib. **Picture 34** shows in detail how the nerve wraps all the way around to the front of the body.

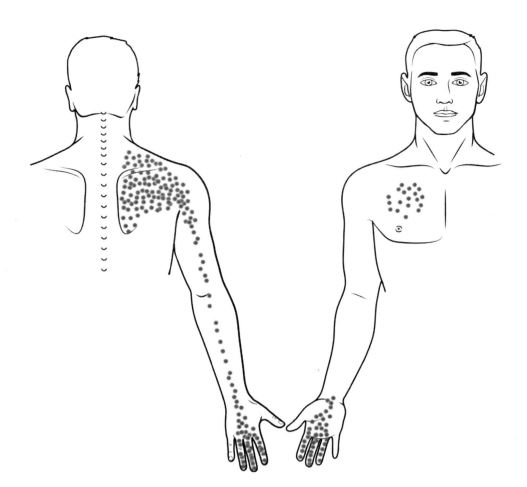

The nerve attaches to all the muscles and skin in the path of each rib. When these nerves are inflamed, this type of pain can mimic a pulled muscle in the rib cage, a broken rib, kidney stones, or a problem with your shoulder blade. It even can feel like you have a hernia because the pain from the thoracic nerves can wrap around to the groin. Read Chapter 11 if you are experiencing pain in the thoracic area of your back.

You may have been told that the MRI of your spine does not show the disc pressing on the nerve, whether it is in the cervical, thoracic, or lumbar spine. Therefore, the pain that you are experiencing cannot possibly be coming from the nerves of the spine. This is totally untrue. It is frequently overlooked that the MRI is usually taken while patients are lying down, and therefore it may not show the whole picture. When you are in a sitting or standing position, rather than lying down, the weight of your body or gravity is pressing on top of the disc, and the disc can protrude more and push against the nerve, a condition that the MRI can miss. In the past twenty years, I have treated many patients with a minimally invasive procedure using local anesthetic and steroids—even when the MRI did not show an obvious problem—and afterward the pain went away. Ensure that you do not lose sight of the clinical picture and start making decisions just by what an MRI shows (or doesn't show).

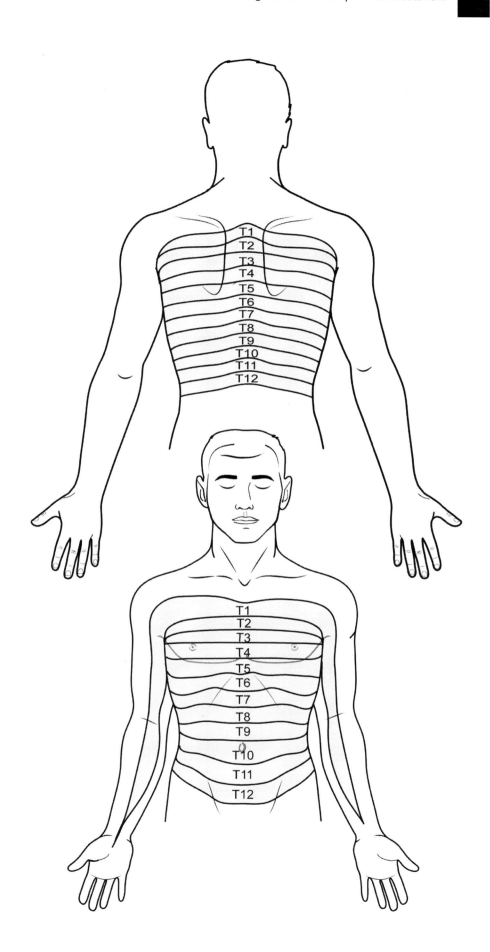

PICTURE 33

Areas of the body that will be painful when specific thoracic nerves are inflamed.

Thoracic nerve

Spinal cord

Vertebra

Disc

Sternum

Spinal nerve

Rib

Lateral branches of
thoracic nerve

Thoracic nerve

The thoracic nerve
starts in the back of
the spine and wraps
all the way around to
the front of the body.

NERVE PAIN

1. Nerve pain can create pain in various parts of the body, with most pain created by nerves in the neck, termed the cervical nerves, or nerves in the lower back, termed the lumbar nerves. You also can have nerve pain in the mid-back that is created by the thoracic nerves.

2. The same cervical, lumbar, and thoracic nerves can create pain, numbness, or weakness.

3. The cervical nerves when inflamed can create pain in the neck, shoulder, and/or arm, or any combination of these three areas. For example, you may notice pain only in the neck at times, and other times you may have neck and shoulder pain, with numbness in the arm. All these conditions can be caused by the same nerve in the neck.

4. The lumbar nerves create pain in the back, hip, buttock, groin, and anywhere in the leg muscles. These nerves can also cause numbness and weakness in different areas at different times. You may notice back pain with numbness in the leg, all coming from the same nerve.

5. The thoracic or mid-back nerves will create pain in the middle of the back, which includes all the areas from between the shoulder blades down to the waistline. This type of pain can wrap around to the front of the body as each one of these nerves is attached to the bottom of the ribs. Therefore, thoracic nerve pain can occur in the shoulder blades, ribs, chest, abdomen, or even groin.

6. Nerve pain can come from the nerve being irritated by the disc or from a narrowing of the hole on the *side* of the spine (foraminal stenosis), or it can be the result of the narrowing of the hole in the *center* canal (spinal stenosis).

7. Pain from the nerve being inflamed due to a disc herniation or foraminal stenosis on the *side* of the vertebrae will create pain that occurs with different positions compared to *central* spinal stenosis.

8. Trying to differentiate these two types of pain is essential, as the treatment, exercises, and even surgery are quite different. The majority of cases of central stenosis pertain to the lumbar spine, but this problem also can occur in the thoracic and cervical areas of the spine.

CHAPTER 3

How to Diagnose Your Pain

THE REASON FOR DIAGNOSIS INSTEAD OF NARCOTICS

I could have written two separate chapters on why you should find a diagnosis before being treated, as well as how not to become a chronic pain patient, but these two topics are intertwined. Before I start to talk about diagnosing and treating neck, mid-back, and lower back pain, I should repeat something that I said earlier in the book.

Most patients with spine pain will get better in the first four to six weeks no matter what they do. Eighty percent of people with acute onset spine pain will improve whether they take medications, use physical therapy, receive chiropractic care, get injections, or just sit around. The human body will correct the situation by eliminating the inflammation and therefore the pain. During this time, patients should do whatever makes them feel better while the body is taking care of itself. You just need to make sure you do not do things that create more pain. This is where a physical therapist or chiropractor may be able to help you. The idea of "working through the pain" is nonsense. Do not do activities that create pain: all that does is aggravate the problem. Chapter 17 will teach you about body mechanics and positions and show you exercises to do in order to manage your pain.

It may be time to find out why you are hurting if you still are having discomfort, and the pain is not getting much better, after four to six weeks since the start of your pain. If you were put on narcotics during your initial onset of pain, that regimen needs to come to an end quickly. Continuing to take narcotic pain medications so that you can mask the pain will lead to a problem called "tolerance" to pain medication. This means that the longer you are on the narcotics, the more narcotics you will need to achieve the same level of relief. Taking narcotics for a long period of time will also increase your sensitivity to pain, which will aggravate the situation.

Let me repeat: *First*, the longer you are on narcotics, the higher the doses of narcotics you will need to keep your same pain under control as your body becomes tolerant of the drugs. *Second*, as you increase your pain medications, your body will become hypersensitive to the same pain you are having. In more than twenty years, I rarely have had a patient on any long-term narcotic pain medication (long-term is more than six weeks). I am not telling you to live in pain. What I am telling you is that if you are not getting better within the first four to six weeks, you need to find the cause of your pain instead of masking it with drugs.

> **Remember: The primary goal should be to locate the specific inflamed structure that is creating the pain. If this can be accomplished, then you will experience minimal chronic pain. Everyday usage of narcotics is needed in only a very few instances.**

This primary goal cannot be taken lightly. It sounds simple but is rarely accomplished, because many medical practitioners attempt to treat pain as a disease and not just a symptom.

> **Remember: The primary reason that patients continue with pain, even though they may have received many types of treatments, is that the exact structure that was creating the pain was never located and treated properly!**

The following examples will illustrate these points. A patient has a herniated disc in her neck and has had headaches and pain in the back of her shoulder for years. Instead of having a minimally invasive diagnostic procedure in which an anti-inflammatory medication is placed in the area of the disc herniation, she receives trigger point injections or Botox injections into the shoulder and neck. Because the pain keeps coming back, she starts on narcotics. Another patient has a herniated disc in his lumbar spine that is creating pain going down into the buttock. Instead of having the disc treated, he is diagnosed with sacroiliac joint syndrome and receives a series of injections in the sacroiliac joint. Because the pain keeps coming back, he is put on narcotics.

Locating the exact problem and then treating it may sound difficult, but it really is not. I wrote this book for one purpose: to help patients diagnose their *own* problem so that they can have it treated properly and *not* live on narcotics or in pain.

THE PAIN DIAGRAM—THE FIRST STEP IN FINDING OUT WHY YOU HURT

The first thing I have patients do when they come to see me is to draw on a picture of the human body to show me exactly where they feel pain, tingling, or numbness. **Picture 35** is the same as the first picture I showed you in this book (Picture 1).

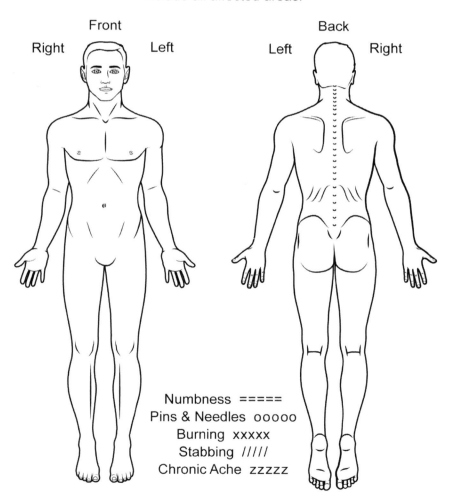

Pain Diagram
Mark the areas on your body where you feel the
described sensations. Use appropriate symbol.
Mark areas of radiation.
Include all affected areas.

Front   Back

Right   Left   Left   Right

Numbness =====
Pins & Needles ooooo
Burning xxxxx
Stabbing /////
Chronic Ache zzzzz

Estimate the severity of your pain (Choose one number)

0 No Pain
1 Mild Pain
2-3 Moderate Pain

4-5 Moderate to Severe Pain
6-7 Severe Pain
8-9 Intensely Severe Pain
10 Most Severe Pain

PICTURE 35

Pain diagram.

After the patient fills out the pain diagram, I match it to the pictures of the spine (Pictures 2, 3, and 5) that show the areas of the body where specific nerves, discs, and facets create pain. This one exercise is key to locating the problem that is creating the patient's pain.

Why do I not just prescribe an MRI at this point? Because an MRI shows the degeneration in your spine; it does not tell you where you hurt. Most areas of degeneration do not create pain unless they are inflamed. There are no studies that show where pain is located! You should first try to locate the problem creating your pain and then see if there is an area on your MRI that would match the problem.

Go ahead and fill out the pain diagram. Mark wherever you have pain or numbness. Then find the section below that matches your area of discomfort.

The Cervical Spine—The Neck, Shoulder, and/or Arm

If you filled in the pain diagram over the area of the neck, shoulder, or arm, then your pain may be coming either from a disc, nerve, or facet joint in your cervical spine. Compare your pain diagram to the illustrations in **Picture 36**. These images show you Pictures 2 and 3 at the same time. The images outside the box show where the cervical nerves create pain over the *surface* of the neck, shoulders, and arms. The image inside the box shows where the *muscles* and *bones* hurt when one of the cervical nerves, discs, or facet joints is inflamed. The pain can be isolated to just the neck, anywhere from the top of the skull all the way down to the base of the neck, or can radiate down into the shoulders. The pain also can go all the way down the arms.

Let's go over a few examples as that is the easiest way to show you how I use these pictures. Let's say you have pain in the area of the shoulder blade and also going down your arm. Here is a picture of what your pain diagram may look like **(Picture 37)**.

If you look at the images *outside* of the box in Picture 36, as well as the one inside the box, you should be able to figure out which cervical nerve, facet, or disc is creating your pain. For example, the C7 nerve creates pain in the back of the shoulder blade as well as pain, numbness, and tingling down the arm. So if you get an MRI of your neck and it shows that you have a large disc herniation pressing on the C4 nerve, and a small disc herniation pressing up against the C7 nerve, which one is probably creating your pain? Which one are you going to treat? The answer is the C7 nerve because it matches where your pain is. Do you see why it is important not to use only the MRI to make decisions?

Let's look at another pain diagram of the neck **(Picture 38)**.

Now compare it to **Picture 39**. As you can see, it matches the C3-C4 level. It could be the disc, facet joint, or nerve that is creating your pain, but you know which level your pain is coming from.

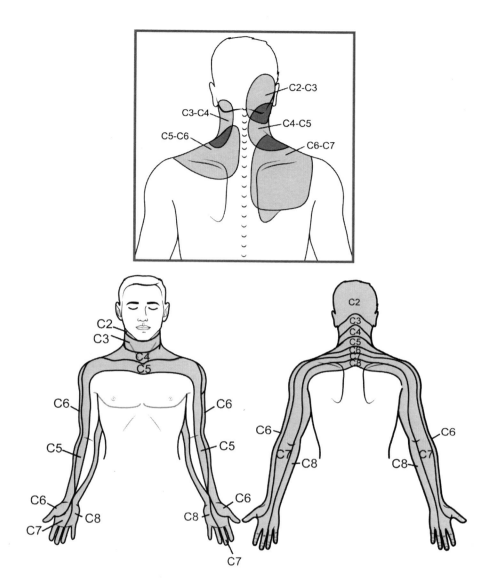

PICTURE 36

The areas of the neck, shoulders, and arms that can hurt from inflammation of specific nerves of the cervical spine.

If you had an MRI done for left-sided upper neck pain and it showed that you had a large disc herniation at C6-C7 and a small arthritic facet joint at C3-C4 on the left, which one are you going to treat? The answer is the C3-C4 facet on the left because that is where your pain is. *Use the MRI only to confirm the problem.* Using this information, you can now look at Chapters 8, 9, and 10 to find more information about your neck, arm, and shoulder pain.

The Thoracic Spine—The Mid-Back

If you filled in the pain diagram in the mid-back area, then your pain is probably due to an inflamed disc, nerve, or joint in the thoracic spine. Picture 34 shows how each thoracic nerve is attached to the bottom of a rib, which is why pain from the thoracic spine can wrap around your body. For example, the T5 nerve starts in the middle of the back and wraps all the way around to the front of the chest **(Picture 40)**.

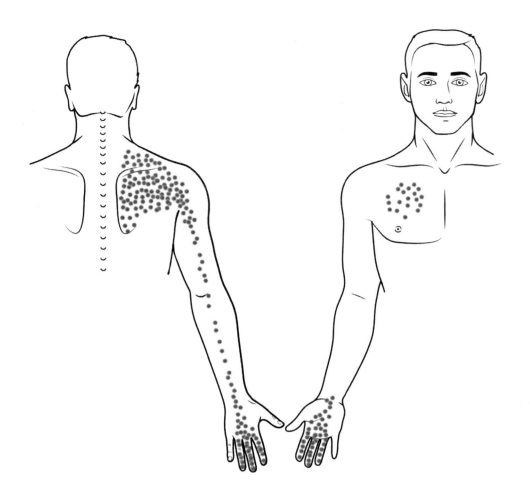

Areas of the body that can hurt when the C7 nerve is inflamed.

The nerves of the thoracic spine can create pain anywhere from the bottom of the neck all the way to the upper back, and they all wrap around to the front of the body. The pain may be anywhere along the path of the thoracic nerve as it does not have to wrap all the way around to the front of the body. I have seen patients with pain in their breast, shoulder blade, kidney area, and even the groin area that was due to an inflamed thoracic nerve. Patients with a thoracic disc herniation and nerve pain may feel like they have a kidney stone, a pulled muscle in their ribs, or even a lung condition as it may hurt to breathe. Chapter 11 provides more information about thoracic disc, nerve, and facet pain.

The Lumbar Spine—The Lower Back, Hip, Groin, Buttock, and/or Leg

If you filled in your lower back, hip, groin, buttock, or leg on the pain diagram, then your pain is probably coming from the lumbar spine. I am going to show you three pictures that you can match to your pain diagram. If your pain is primarily in your back, **Picture 41** is the picture to compare your

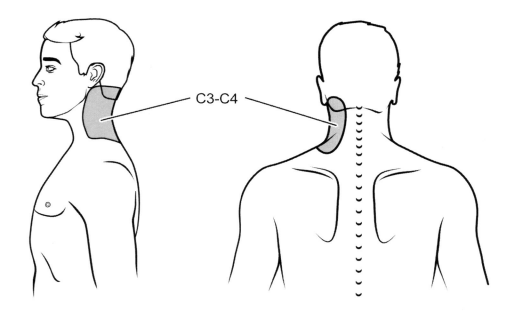

PICTURE 38

Left-sided upper neck pain due to a disc, nerve, or facet joint at the C3-C4 level.

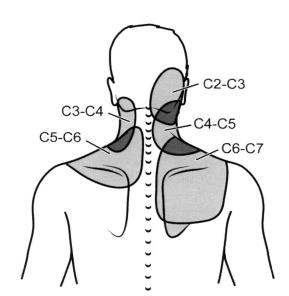

PICTURE 39

The specific areas of the body that can hurt because of an inflamed cervical nerve, disc, or facet.

pain diagram to. The picture shows where each level of disc or facet joint can create pain. If your pain is *only* in your lower back, you are usually looking at a disc or facet as the cause of your pain. The disc or the facet can also create pain radiating into the hip or down the leg, but it *never* goes past the knee. So if the L5-S1 disc is inflamed, it will create pain in the lower back and down into the side of the lower buttock. If the L3-L4 facet joint is inflamed, it will cause pain in the upper part of the lower back. Once you have located the level of your pain by comparing this picture to your pain diagram, you can turn to the chapter that best describes your pain, as that will help you determine whether it is your disc or facet joint that is creating your pain. Chapters 4, 5, and 6 will give you information about back pain.

The specific areas of the body that can hurt because of inflamed thoracic nerves.

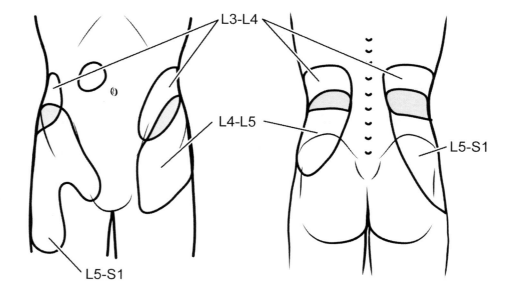

PICTURE 41

Areas of lower back
pain when a specific
lumbar disc or facet
is inflamed.

The second image shows where you would feel pain on *the* surface of the
body when one of the *nerves* in the lumbar spine is inflamed (**Picture 42**).
These nerves start in the lumbar spine and go down into the area of the back,
hip, buttock, groin, and leg. The pain can be anywhere along the path of the
nerve. For instance, the L4 nerve when inflamed may create pain only in the
side of the hip, or it may cause pain starting in the back and then go down
the side of the hip to the shin. Similarly, the L5 nerve may create pain only
in your back, buttock, or the side of your leg or a combination of all three.

The next picture shows you the *muscles* and *bones* that the same lumbar
nerves go to (**Picture 43**). I want to point out two important things in this
picture when you compare it to Picture 42. The first is that *different* lumbar
nerves go to the *same* area. In Picture 42, the *skin* of the groin area is covered
by the L1 and L2 nerves. In Picture 43, you can see that the *muscles* and *bones*
of the groin are covered by the L4, L5, and S1 nerves. If you have groin pain
and look only at Picture 42, you would not realize that the L4 and L5 nerves
also can create groin pain. The second thing to see in these pictures is that
the *same* nerve goes to *different* areas. For example, Picture 42 shows that the
L4 nerve goes to the area of *skin* on the side of the hip and the leg. Picture 43
shows that the same L4 nerve goes to the *muscles* of the lower buttock area. If
you have pain in the lower buttock area and look only at Picture 42, you would
think that only inflammation of the S1 or S2 nerve could create that type of
pain, instead of realizing that the L4 nerve can also create lower buttock pain.

So you always should combine both pictures to show the areas of skin,
muscles, and bones each nerve covers. **Picture 44** shows all the areas that the
L4 nerve covers (skin, muscles, and bones.) The pain from the nerve can be
anywhere along the path of the nerve. The same nerve may create *only* back
pain, hip pain, leg pain, groin pain, shin pain, buttock pain, or groin pain, or it
may cause pain in some combination of all these different areas.

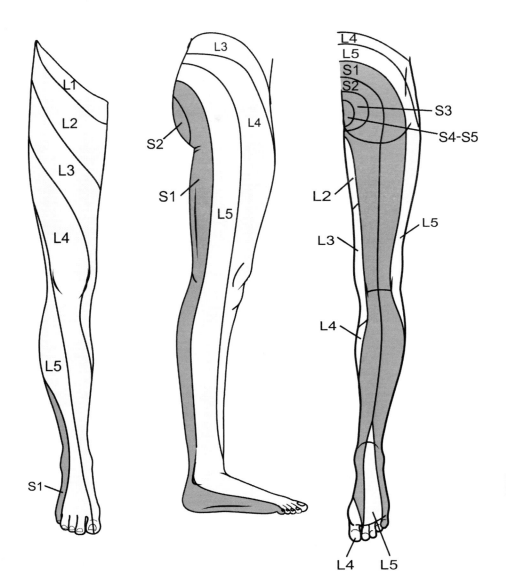

The areas of the body that can hurt because of specific lumbar nerves.

Why do I keep showing these same pictures in each chapter? Why not let your medical practitioner tell you what is going on? Because it appears at times that these pictures are a big secret that nobody has seen. Many patients have come to see me with groin pain and their MRI showed a disc herniation at L4-L5 pressing on the L4 nerve. But nobody ever told them that the L4 nerve could create their groin pain. I have had even more patients with buttock pain who have been diagnosed with piriformis syndrome and sacroiliac joint pain that did not get better with therapy and injections, because the medical practitioners did not realize that the L4 and L5 nerves in the lumbar spine go to the piriformis muscle and the sacroiliac joint, which are both in the buttock area. There was nothing wrong with the piriformis muscle or sacroiliac joint. The problem was an inflamed nerve in the lumbar spine creating pain in the piriformis muscle and/or sacroiliac joint. Once the lumbar nerve was treated, the piriformis pain and the sacroiliac joint pain went away.

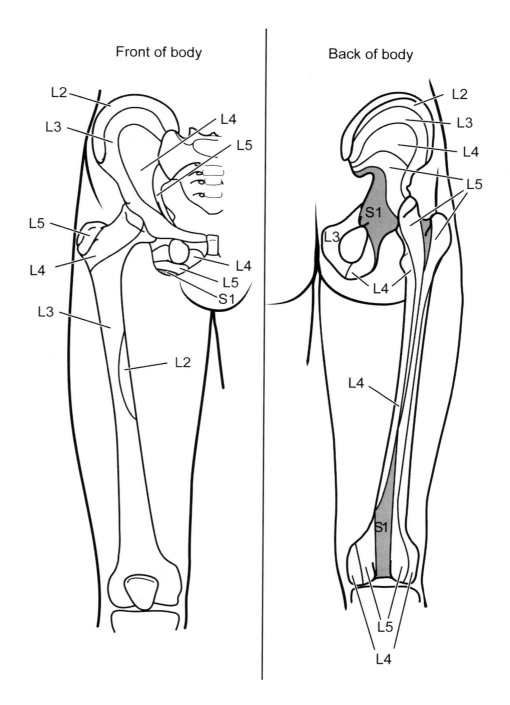

Front of body

Back of body

PICTURE 43

Inflamed lumbar nerves can create pain in the muscles and bones of the hip, buttock, and pelvis.

Another common example is pain in the side of the hip. Is it bursitis of the hip? Or is it due to inflammation of one of your lumbar nerve roots? If you look at Picture 42 and Picture 43, what you will see is that the skin and muscle of the side of your hip are covered by the L4 and L5 nerves. So if the side of your hip is painful and the muscle over the bursa is very tender, do not forget that the source may be an inflamed L4 or L5 nerve, not bursitis of the hip. Even if your back or leg does not hurt! Remember, an inflamed lumbar nerve will not always create pain down your leg. It could create pain just in the groin, buttock, or the side of your hip.

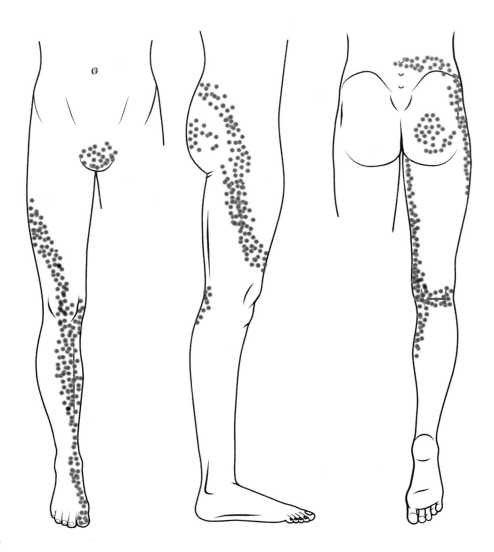

The areas of the body that may be painful when the L4 nerve is inflamed.

You may be wondering why I do not just order an MRI to find the problem creating your pain. For one reason: *the MRI cannot diagnose pain. It just tells you what is degenerated.* We are all going to have degenerated structures as we age, but most of these structures will never create pain unless they become inflamed. You can use the MRI to help you once you have narrowed down the problem. For example, if you have pain in the side of your hip and you have an MRI done that shows a large disc herniation at L2-L3 and a smaller one at L4-L5, which one would you treat? Since you filled out a pain diagram and you have looked at Pictures 42 and 43, you know that the smaller L4-L5 disc is creating your problem. *Use the MRI to confirm a diagnosis, not to determine the diagnosis.*

Why do I spend so much time trying to *find the specific problem creating your pain*? If you do not find the problem creating your pain, your pain will not go away. And if your pain does not go away, then you may have to take narcotic pain medications to manage your pain. And at some point you will become addicted to the narcotic pain medications. Instead, why not find the problem, treat or fix the problem, and learn about body mechanics and exercise so that your pain does not recur as often?

After reading this chapter, you now know the area of your spine that is probably creating your pain, if your pain is coming from your spine. Chapter 2 gave you information about the different structures in your spine that can create your pain. I suggest that you should now turn to Part II of this book and find the chapter and/or chapters that most closely resemble your pain. Read all the chapters that may pertain to your pain. For example, if your neck and arm hurt, read both Chapters 9 and 10. You are getting closer to finding out why you hurt!

SUMMARY

1. Draw the areas of your pain on a pain diagram (Picture 35).

2. Compare this diagram with the pictures of the body that show where different levels of the spine create pain.

3. If your pain is in your neck, shoulder, and/or arm, use Pictures 36 and 39.

4. If your pain is in your mid-back, use Picture 40.

5. If your pain is in your lower back, hip, groin, buttock, or leg, use Pictures 41, 42, and 43.

6. Next, read the chapters in Part II that most resemble the type of pain you are having.

7. You can then consider obtaining an MRI to help you confirm a diagnosis.

8. Read Chapter 16, which will give you information about minimally invasive procedures that are both diagnostic and therapeutic.

9. Read Chapter 17, which suggests exercises to use to minimize your pain, teaches you about posture and body mechanics to keep your pain from returning, and shows how to strengthen your body without aggravating your spine.

PART II

Common Complaints

My Back and/or Leg Hurts When I Sit, but Feels Better When I Walk

The two structures that create most back and leg pain when you sit are an inflamed lumbar disc or nerve (**Picture 45**). A herniated or bulging disc can inflame the nerve, or the nerve may become irritated and painful if the hole where the nerve exits becomes narrowed due to arthritis. This is called foraminal stenosis.

Picture 46 shows the area of the back and leg that each nerve coming out of the lumbar spine covers. You can match your pain with this picture to give you an idea of which nerve is creating your discomfort. You may feel pain anywhere along the path of the nerve. The pain could be just in your back, just in the side of your hip, just in your leg, or a combination of these.

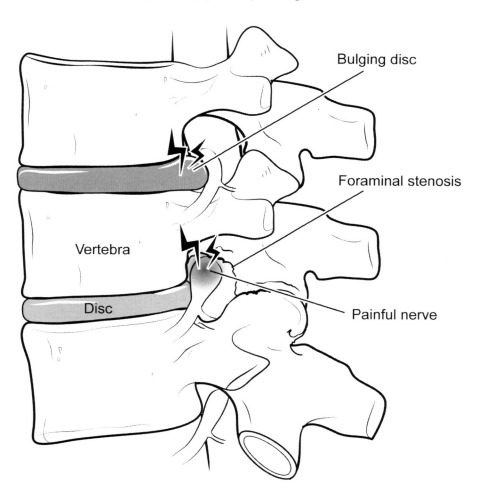

Bulging disc

Foraminal stenosis

Vertebra

Disc

Painful nerve

PICTURE 45

Disc herniation or foraminal stenosis can create an inflamed lumbar nerve.

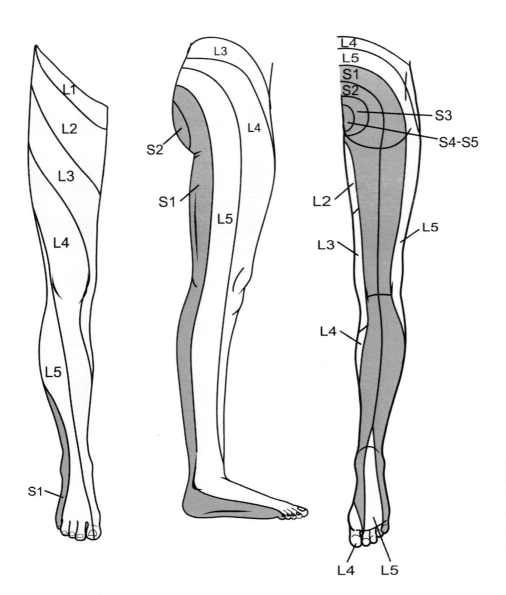

The lumbar disc can also create pain due to the *inside* of the disc becoming inflamed. There are nerves that are located in the outer portion of the *inside* of the disc. This area is called the annulus. **Picture 47** shows two ways in which a disc can create back pain. The top image shows a disc herniation inflaming a nerve, which can create back pain. The bottom image shows an inflammation of a tear inside the disc with *no* disc herniation, but because the annulus is inflamed the disc will create back pain.

As we age, all discs will have tears, but most of them will not become inflamed. If the inside of the disc becomes inflamed, it can create back pain when you sit for an extended period of time or bend forward from the waist. The inside of the disc can create pain without the disc being herniated. So even though an MRI may not show a disc herniation, you still can have severe back pain resulting from the inflammation *inside* the disc. **Picture 48** shows where you would feel pain if the lower lumbar discs are inflamed.

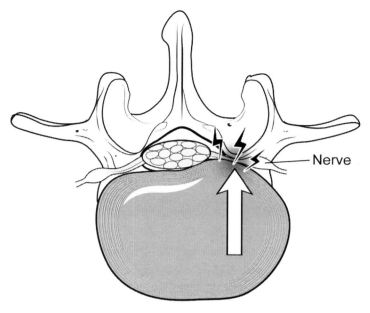

Disc herniation

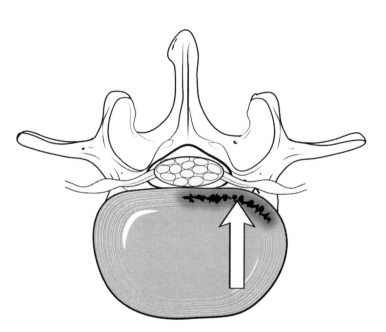

Annular tear

PICTURE 47

(top) A disc herniation and (bottom) an inflamed tear inside the disc with no herniation.

Lower back pain experienced while sitting usually is due to inflammation of the discs and/or the nerves. Identifying the exact source of pain will give you the information you need to eradicate it, ensure that you do the correct exercises to help you recover from the painful occurrence, and enable you to use this information to avoid re-irritating that part of the spine.

If your back hurts while you're in the sitting position but gets better when you walk, it usually points to the disc and/or the nerve as the source of inflammation. The sitting position does two things to the spine. First, it

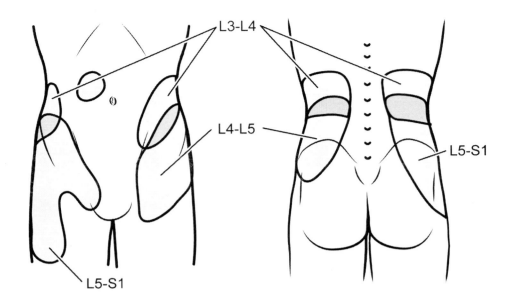

L3-L4

L4-L5

L5-S1

L5-S1

Areas of pain when the lumbar discs are inflamed.

loads the disc in your back because of the pressure of body weight and gravity, which can create back pain if the inflammation is inside the disc or create pain going down the leg if the outer part of the inflamed disc irritates and inflames the nerve. Second, the sitting position creates a stretching of your lumbar nerves as they exit the spine and go down the legs. The stretching of the nerve in the sitting position can aggravate an already inflamed nerve. Therefore, you may notice pain in the back or the leg from prolonged sitting if the nerve is inflamed. **Picture 49** shows how the nerve may stretch and lengthen when you are in a sitting position.

The most common reason that I see patients squirming when they are in the sitting position is disc and/or nerve pain, either because of the inflammation of the outside of the disc inflaming the nerve or the inflammation inside of the disc. This discomfort is increased due to body weight or gravity placing pressure on an inflamed disc or nerve.

Several other body positions will make inflamed disc pain worse. Leaning forward at the waist will increase the pressure in the disc and may increase back pain if the disc is irritated. You may notice that coming up from a sitting to a standing position can increase back pain as your spine straightens because of an inflamed disc. When I walk into an exam room to see a patient, two possible positions make me think that the patient's pain is coming from the disc. First, the patient may be standing or walking around the room and does not like sitting. Second, the patient is either sitting with the back arched or leaning backward to avoid being in pain. These patients do not want to sit with their back straight or leaning forward.

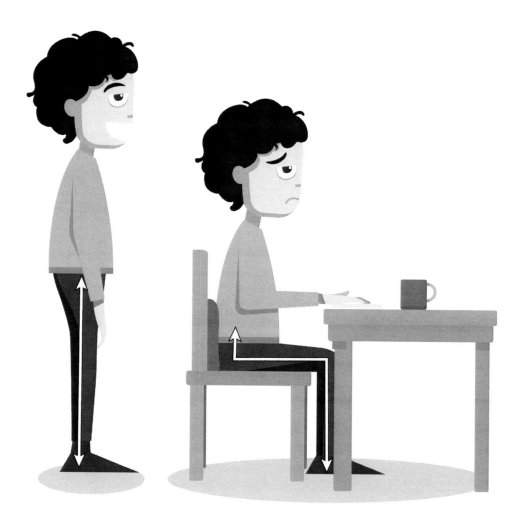

Stretching of the nerve in a sitting position.

Picture 50 shows how the pressure inside a disc increases as you go from a standing position to a sitting position with your back arched, to a sitting position with your back straight, and finally to a leaning-forward position. As you can see, the pressure in the disc increases when you sit with your back straight and keeps getting worse as you lean forward. This is the same reason I encourage patients to work in a standing position, as doing so will decrease the pressure on the disc. If you are sitting, sit up straight or, even better, sit leaning backward.

If you have disc pain, you may notice that while you are sitting, you will use your arms to push down on the arms of the chair or a seat cushion, as that will take pressure off an inflamed disc. This actually is a form of traction, maybe better termed auto-traction.

The other group of patients that has a difficult time when sitting includes patients with nerve or sciatic pain. The outside of the disc actually may inflame the nerve and create the sciatic pain. The sitting position, as noted, can create a pull on the nerve that is relieved by either standing or

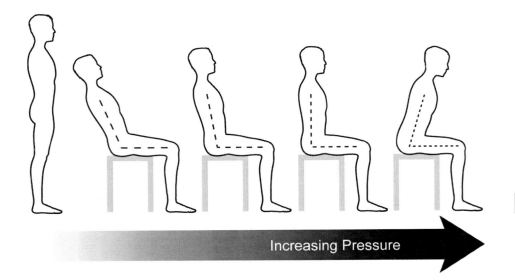

Increasing Pressure

PICTURE 50

Increasing disc
pressure depending
on how you sit.

straightening the leg. Patients with an inflamed nerve feel increased pain while they are driving, as that position adds pressure on the disc as well as stretches the nerve, which in turn will aggravate the nerve and create discomfort. Patients with an inflamed nerve who have to sit will try to sit on the buttock opposite the side that is hurting and will try to straighten the leg out to decrease the stretch on the nerve.

SUMMARY

1. Pain in the lower back or the leg in the sitting position usually points to inflammation of the disc or nerve.

2. Most patients feel better when they are walking around because that position will take the pressure off the disc and decrease the stretch of the inflamed nerve that occurs in the sitting position.

3. Read Chapters 2 and 3 for more information about disc and nerve pain.

4. Chapter 16 provides information on minimally invasive procedures that can be used to diagnose and treat this problem.

5. Chapter 17 will give you information about therapy and exercises for disc and nerve pain.

CHAPTER 5

My Back Keeps Me from Sleeping at Night and/or It Hurts to Stand in One Place

One of the most common structures that create lower back pain when you are sleeping or standing in one place is the facet, commonly called the joint. As you may recall, the facets are located in the *back* of the spine (**Picture 51**).

Because the facet joint is in the back of the spine, anything that creates an arch in your back, such as bending backward, standing in one place, or lying down on your back, will create increased pressure in the joints and create pain if the joint is inflamed. Picture 51 shows that when you bend forward, which is called flexion, your facet joints open up, and as you bend backward, or arch your back, which is called extension, the facet joints press on each other. If the facets are inflamed, the standing position alone can create significant pain. This is because your spine normally goes into an arched or extension position when you are standing, thus creating pressure on the facets. Patients with facet pain usually feel much better when they are walking because this movement allows for more space between the facet joints and therefore creates less pain.

The arching of the back, which gives patients with disc pain relief, makes facet pain worse. Patients with facet joint pain tend to hurt more at night when they are lying on their back, because the spine naturally goes into an arched position, which can create an irritation of the facet joints. You may also notice that sleeping on your stomach is uncomfortable if your facet joints are inflamed, because this position will also create an arch in your spine. Usually these patients tend to lie on their sides and sleep in a fetal position so that their facets do not touch each other.

You will *not* have leg pain if your back pain is due to inflamed facets. You can have back pain or buttock pain, or even pain that wraps around to the front of your groin, but the pain will never go past the back of the knee. **Picture 52** shows where the facet joints most commonly create pain in the lower back. For example, when the L5-S1 facet joint is inflamed, it can create pain into the lower buttock, the hip, and possibly the groin area. Leg pain should tell you that your pain is coming from the nerve, not the facet.

The facet can become enlarged and arthritic, and subsequently narrow the hole where the nerve comes through by the facet (**Picture 53**). If that occurs, then the patient will have *nerve* pain, not *facet* pain. I see countless patients who have leg pain and are treated as if they have facet pain.

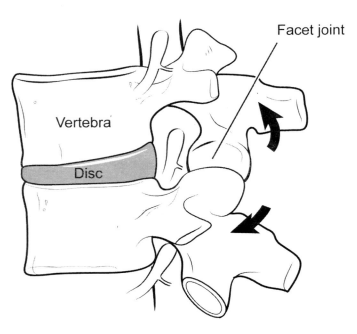

Facet joint

Vertebra

Disc

Flexion (bending forward)

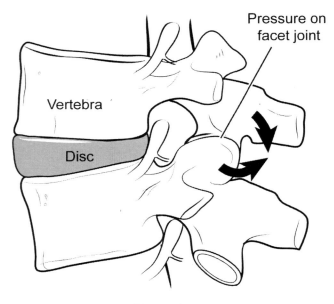

Pressure on
facet joint

Vertebra

Disc

Extension
(arching the back or bending backward)

PICTURE 51

Facet joints open
when you bend
forward and press
on each other when
you bend backward.

Usually patients with facet pain feel better throughout the day because their back is not in an extension position and they can sit slumped forward to keep the pressure off the facets. Interestingly, when I walk into an exam room, I will notice that a patient who has facet pain will be sitting slightly bent over to take the pressure off the joints. Remember, this is the opposite of the patient who has disc pain, who usually sits in an arched position to avoid placing pressure on the disc.

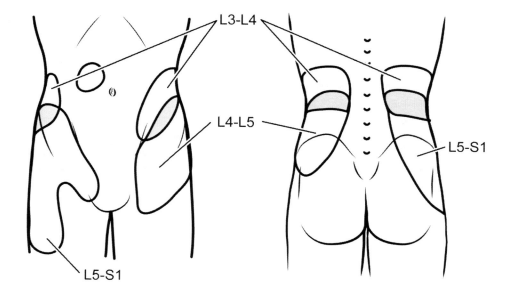

PICTURE 52

Different areas where you will feel pain depending on which lumbar facet is inflamed.

Patients may notice back pain during the day if they are performing activities like swimming or yoga that involve arching or twisting their back. Patients with inflamed facets may experience pain when they get up from a sitting position or come down a flight of stairs, as they have to extend their back to do that. As mentioned, if your facets are inflamed, your back will hurt when you stand in one place, but it feels better when you walk. Most people will lean forward slightly when they stand or walk, which in turn opens up the facets. Keeping a straight back when standing creates pressure on the facets, and if they are inflamed, this position will create pain. Once you start walking, however, the pressure on the joints decreases as you lean forward, and so will your pain.

If you have facet pain, it will hurt if you are sitting in a chair with a lumbar support, as that creates an arch in your spine, and therefore it will irritate the inflamed facets. I know this may sound strange, but a chair with a lumbar support is *not* good for someone with facet pain. This shows you how essential it is to know what structure is creating your pain before you modify your office to become more ergonomically correct. A standing desk is great for someone with sciatic nerve or disc pain, but it is not good for someone with facet or stenosis pain.

Another problem in the spine that can mimic the pain that comes from inflammation of the facets is spinal stenosis. Spinal stenosis, which is a narrowing of the spinal canal, and inflamed lumbar facets both can create discomfort at night if you sleep on your back or stomach, and can increase pain in your back if you stand in one place. Chapter 6 discusses spinal stenosis, but I raise this issue now as the treatment and therapy options are quite different between the two. Patients with spinal stenosis have a few symptoms that

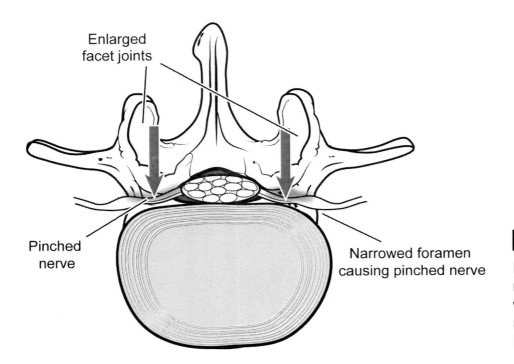

Enlarged facet joints

Pinched nerve

Narrowed foramen causing pinched nerve

Enlarged facets can narrow the foramen, which can pinch the nerve and create leg pain.

usually are not seen in patients with facet pain. Patients with spinal stenosis can have cramps in their legs at night or pain going down their legs, and the back and leg pain will get worse with walking. Patients with facet pain will never have leg pain or cramps, and their pain gets better when they walk.

SUMMARY

1. Back pain from inflamed lumbar facet joints can keep you from sleeping at night or cause pain when you first get out of bed.

2. Standing in one place will also make facet pain worse, and you will notice that the pain gets better when you walk.

3. Lumbar facets never create leg pain.

4. The facet joint may become enlarged and irritate the nerve that runs by it, but then the nerve should be treated and not the facet joint.

5. The pain from facet pain and spinal stenosis are similar as both create pain when you sleep or when you stand.

6. The difference is that facet pain never goes down the leg and gets better when you walk.

7. Pain from spinal stenosis will get even more painful as you walk and commonly creates leg pain and cramps.

8. You can have pain from both the facets and spinal stenosis at the same time.

9. Chapters 2 and 3 provide more information about facet pain.

10. Chapter 6 talks about spinal stenosis.

11. Chapter 16 provides details on the minimally invasive procedures that can diagnose and treat facet and spinal stenosis pain.

12. Chapter 17 gives you information about therapy and exercises for lumbar facet joint pain and spinal stenosis.

CHAPTER 6

My Back and/or Legs Hurt When I Stand or Walk, but Feel Better When I Sit

Back and leg pain are two of the most common complaints that I see in my practice. When all humans stand or walk, the spine straightens and the spinal canal narrows. This position creates a smaller space in your spinal canal compared with when you are sitting. This usually has no effect on the nerves in the center of the canal, and it creates no symptoms because the spinal canal has plenty of room to accommodate these changes—unless you have spinal stenosis. Spinal stenosis is a combination of protruding discs, thickening ligaments, and enlarged joints that creates a narrow spinal canal (**Picture 54**).

When the spinal stenosis creates inflammation inside the canal, it causes characteristic symptoms. If you have this type of pain, you will notice that as you walk, your pain usually gets worse. When you stop and sit down, you feel dramatic relief. The pain can be just in the back, or it can be only in the legs, or it can be a combination of the two. You may also notice that the pain gets worse when you stand erect or bend backward and that the pain lessens when you bend forward, because that opens the canal and gives the nerves more breathing room. **Picture 55** shows what happens with spinal stenosis if you stand up straight versus bending forward.

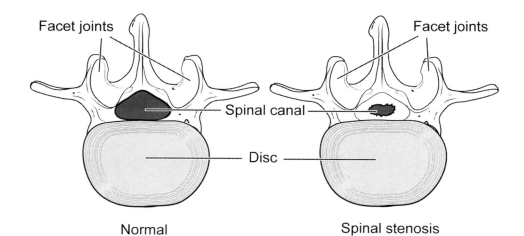

PICTURE 54

Spinal stenosis.

Normal   Spinal stenosis

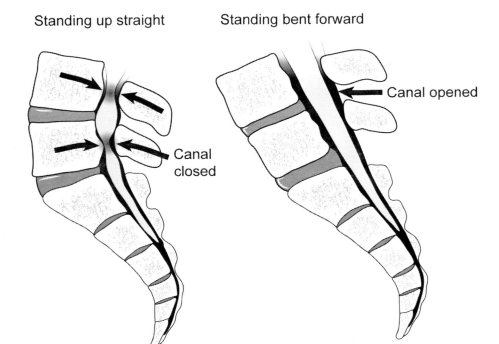

Standing up straight

Standing bent forward

Canal opened

Canal closed

The spinal canal opens when you bend forward.

One of the first questions I ask patients who appear to have pain from spinal stenosis is whether they tend to hang on to a shopping cart in the grocery store, as demonstrated in **Picture 56**. This position allows them to bend forward while shopping, which opens up their canal and gives them some relief.

If you have spinal stenosis and you do not like to hang out in grocery stores, you may tend to bend forward when you walk and lean on things to open up your spinal canal. Family members may tell you to straighten up, because they do not realize that walking bent over allows you to feel better, because it gives your spinal canal more room. I advise patients with severe spinal stenosis to use a walker with a seat on it. The walker does two things: it allows you to walk bent over, thus providing the spinal canal with more room for the nerves, and gives you a place to sit down for several minutes every half hour or so, which will keep the spinal stenosis from becoming inflamed.

> **Remember: If you have been treated for spinal stenosis and are starting to feel better, you should learn to sit down every half hour for about five minutes, even if you have no pain. This will keep the nerves inside your spinal canal from becoming inflamed.**

Just because your pain is gone after it is treated with a minimally invasive procedure does not mean that there is any change in the narrowing of the spinal canal. The only thing that has changed is that the inflammation is gone, thus decreasing your pain. The easiest way to keep the nerves in the area

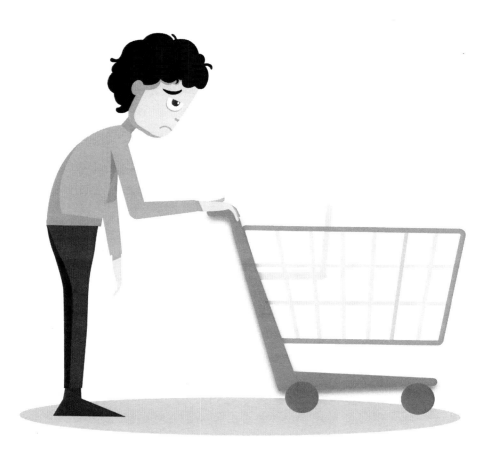

PICTURE 56

The shopping cart sign.

of narrowing from becoming inflamed again is to frequently sit down *before* you start to hurt. Once you start hurting and you start sitting down, it will be difficult to eliminate the inflammation without having that area treated with steroids. Chapter 16 provides information on the treatment for spinal stenosis.

If you have spinal stenosis, you may notice that you have a problem sleeping on your back with your spine straightened. This position also narrows your spine for the same reason as when you are standing up straight. Patients with spinal stenosis tell me their worst time is when they first get out of bed with a stiff and painful back, but their pain gets better throughout the day as long as they are not on their feet a lot. You may notice that you feel much better if you sleep on your side curled up in a fetal position, because this position keeps the spinal canal open. I encourage patients to keep a pillow between their legs and even stuff a pillow behind their back so that they will not roll onto their back while they are sleeping. If you really like sleeping on your back, sleep with the head of the bed raised about thirty to forty degrees, by using an electric bed frame or a wedge—or sleep in a recliner instead of a bed. This position will give your spinal canal more room and keep it from becoming inflamed.

People with spinal stenosis may notice that they have cramps and pain in their legs at night, especially if they sleep on their back, because the straight spine position creates a narrowing of the canal and squeezes the nerves in the spine that go down the legs. A lot of patients with spinal stenosis who thought their leg pain was due to restless leg syndrome or neuropathy notice that their leg symptoms get much better once their spinal stenosis is treated.

If you have spinal stenosis, you may notice that your feet swell. This swelling can be due to the inflammation of the nerves in the lumbar spine from the stenosis. Once the inflammation subsides, the swelling in your feet also goes away.

I always diagnose painful spinal stenosis by what the patient tells me. This is an essential part of treating spinal stenosis in the lumbar spine. For example, if a practitioner tells you that you merely have arthritis in your back, but you cannot walk far without hurting and you feel a lot better when you sit down, you probably have spinal stenosis. In this case, the large "arthritic" facet joints are probably narrowing the canal, as seen in Picture 54. Another example is if you have been told that you have "spondylolisthe-sis," which is a fancy term that means one part of your spine has slipped over the other **(Picture 57)**.

Spondylolisthesis is a common finding on MRIs and has no clinical significance if you are not hurting other than you should remember to bend your knees to keep the slipping to a minimum. At times, this slippage can create painful stenosis in the spine; if so, you may notice discomfort when you are walking and will feel much better when you sit down.

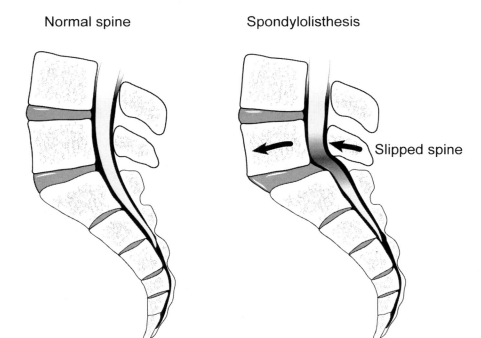

Normal spine   Spondylolisthesis

Slipped spine

PICTURE 57

Spondylolisthesis creating spinal stenosis.

SUMMARY

1. Spinal stenosis is a common problem that affects the fifty-and-over age group.

2. The combination of disc herniations, thickened ligaments, and enlarged facet joints creates a narrowing of the spinal canal, which, when inflamed, can create pain in the back and legs.

3. You will notice that your pain gets worse when you stand and walk, but gets much better when you sit down.

4. You can minimize this discomfort by changing how you do your daily activities.

5. To learn more about spinal stenosis, read Chapter 2.

6. Chapter 16 provides information on the treatment of spinal stenosis.

7. Chapter 17 gives information about therapy and exercises if you have spinal stenosis.

My Hip Hurts

Hip pain is one of the most frequent complaints that patients have. This can be a confusing issue for many patients, because they do not realize that the area they are calling their hip is usually just their buttock muscles and the surrounding muscles of the hip.

The hip joint is actually located in the *front* part of your pelvis, and the closest area on the human body to the hip joint is the groin (**Picture 58**).

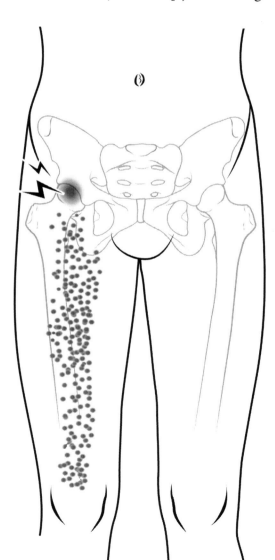

PICTURE 58

Pain in the groin and the front of the leg because of an inflamed hip joint.

Therefore, when patients have pain originating from their hip joint, it is usually groin pain. The pain will start in the groin and can go down the front of the leg, stopping above the knee. If the pain goes past the knee, it usually is coming from a nerve in the spine. Pain from the hip joint *never* goes down the side of the leg or past the knee.

There is no hip joint in most of the buttock area. The only buttock pain that you will have with a hip problem is very *low in the buttock* where the crease of your buttock meets the leg **(Picture 59)**.

Diagnosing pain that actually comes from the hip joint usually can be done clinically on examination. See whether you can cross the leg on the side you think has a hip joint problem over the other leg while in a sitting position, as shown in **Picture 60**. If you cross your leg and notice that you have increased pain in the groin area, your pain may be coming from the hip.

If you are able to cross your leg without having pain in your groin, your pain is probably not coming from your hip.

Most pain in the groin and buttock area is *not* due to the hip, but instead it is due to one of the structures in the lumbar spine. The most common structure that creates pain in the area of the groin and buttock is one of the lumbar nerve roots. As you can see in the left-hand image of **Picture 61**, the L4, L5, and S1 nerves cover the muscles and bones of the groin, and therefore if one of these nerves is inflamed it can create groin pain. The L1 and

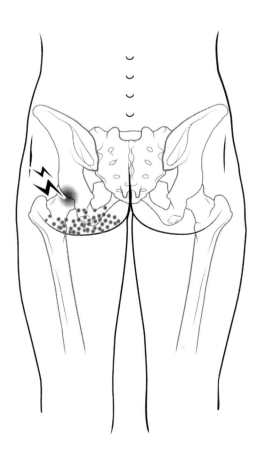

PICTURE 59

Pain in the low buttock when the hip joint is inflamed.

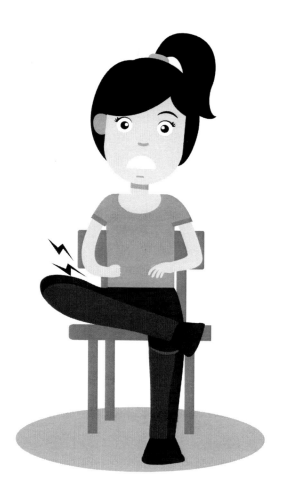

Crossing your leg to see whether it creates groin pain.

L2 nerves can also create groin pain. The right-hand image shows the L3, L4, L5, and S1 nerves that cover the area of the buttock and most commonly create buttock pain.

I have just told you that pain in your buttock area does not usually originate in your hip. But what about the side of your hip? Look at **Picture 62**.

There is a bursa, which is a sac of fluid that decreases the friction between tissues, over this part of the hip. This bursa can become inflamed and therefore create pain. Many patients tell me that they have been diagnosed with bursitis and point to this area. Now I am going to tell you something about this area, just the way I told you about your buttock: *the problem usually is not bursitis,* even if the area feels very tender. This area is usually painful because one of the nerves in the lumbar spine is inflamed as a result of a disc herniation or a narrowing of the spinal canal, which in turn inflames the nerve. **Picture 63** shows that the L3, L4, and L5 nerves cover the side of the hip. When the nerves in the lumbar spine are inflamed, they can create pain over the bursa on the side of your hip.

Many patients who present with pain in their buttock, groin, and the area over the side of the hip actually have a problem with their lumbar spine

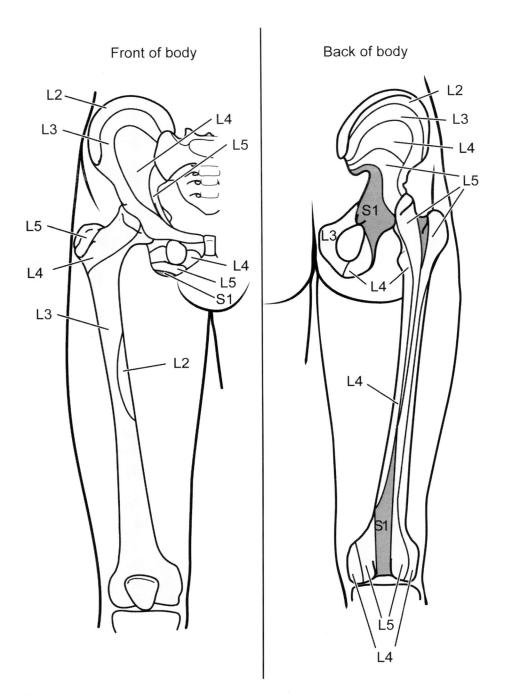

Front of body

Back of body

L2

L3

L4

L5

L5

L4

L3

L2

L4

L5

S1

L2

L3

L4

L5

S1

L3

L4

L5

L4

S1

L5

L4

PICTURE 61

Nerves in the lumbar spine can create groin and buttock pain when they are inflamed.

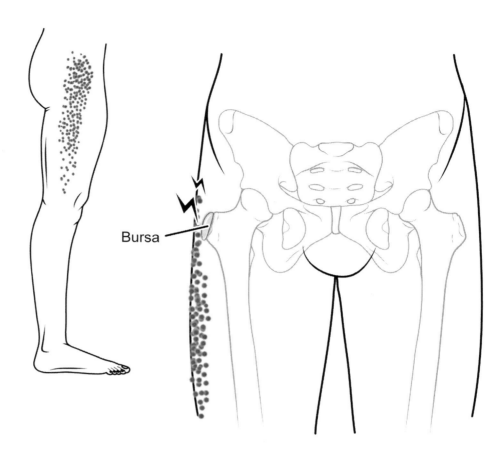

Bursa

PICTURE 62

Bursitis of the hip.

instead of their hip. The pain usually is due to an inflammation from either a herniated disc in the spine, a narrowing of the central canal, or a narrowing of the hole on the side of the spine where the nerve exits. You may notice horrible groin pain, significant tenderness over the area that you think is your hip bursa, and radiation of the pain into the back of the hip and buttock muscles. All this pain can come from your back.

In my clinical practice, it is easy to diagnose whether your "hip" pain is coming from the hip joint. I can use an X-ray machine and put a local anesthetic into the hip joint, and then I will have you immediately walk around and cross your leg over the other one, as I noted earlier. If your pain is gone immediately after I do this, then you know you have a hip problem. If the pain is still there, it means that you probably have a spine issue.

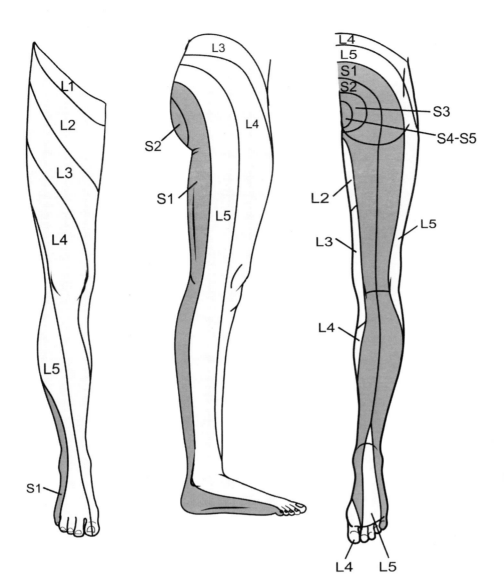

PICTURE 63

Areas of the body where you feel pain when the lumbar nerves are inflamed.

SUMMARY

1. Pain in the area of the hip, groin, and leg usually is due to inflammation of one of the structures of the lumbar spine, whether it is the disc, nerve, or joint, and is not due to the hip joint.

2. Inflammation of the hip joint creates pain only in the groin area, low buttock area, and down the front of the leg to the knee.

3. The pain on the side of the hip is commonly diagnosed as "bursitis." Pain in this area is usually due to one of the lumbar nerves that cover the skin and muscles over the bursa, and not to an inflammation of the bursa of the hip.

4. It is essential to identify the exact structure that is creating your pain!

5. Read Chapters 2 and 3 for more information on the specific nerves that create hip, groin, and buttock pain.

6. Chapter 16 provides information on minimally invasive diagnostic procedures that show you how to diagnose and treat your hip pain.

7. Chapter 17 gives you information about therapy and exercises.

My Shoulder Hurts—I Have Pain Around My Shoulder Blade

Shoulder pain usually is caused by a shoulder problem or by inflammation in one of the structures in the neck. The structure in the neck, whether it is the facet joint, the disc, or the nerve, can create pain in the front or back of the shoulder. I have had episodes of severe shoulder pain that I thought were coming from my shoulder because it hurt to move the shoulder. I later found out the herniated disc in my neck was inflaming a nerve in my spine that goes to my shoulder. Sometimes my pain has been in the front of the shoulder and other times it feels like I have an ice pick in my shoulder blade.

Pain that originates from problems in the cervical spine can create discomfort either in the front or back of the shoulder. You may feel sure the pain is originating in your shoulder because it hurts to move your shoulder and you may not have any neck pain. However, the structures in the neck (disc, facet joint, or nerve) can create pain from the top of the shoulder all the way down to the bottom of the shoulder blade, depending on which disc, facet joint, or nerve is involved.

Look at **Picture 64**. If you look at the two images *outside* the box, you will see where each nerve in the cervical spine goes. If you follow the C5, C6, and C7 nerves all the way from the neck down past the shoulder, you will see that these nerves are the ones that primarily cover the *skin* over most of the shoulder. If you look at the image *inside* the box, you see the *muscles* of the shoulder that the nerves, facets, and discs go to. You will see that the disc, facet joint, or nerve of the C4-C5, C5-C6, and C6-C7 levels of the spine can create pain in the back of the shoulder all the way down to the shoulder blade. This means that the disc, nerve, or facet joint at each of these levels can create pain in the area shown in these pictures if they are inflamed.

You may or may not have neck pain at the same time as you are having shoulder pain, even though the shoulder pain is produced by a nerve, joint, or disc in the neck. The same goes for arm pain. You may have shoulder pain that is created by a nerve in your neck, but have no arm pain. Or you might have numbness and tingling in the arm along with your shoulder pain, as the C5, C6, or C7 nerve can create both. The pain from the cervical nerve can get worse when moving the shoulder, or it may get better at times if you raise your arm over your head. You also may notice that your shoulder pain

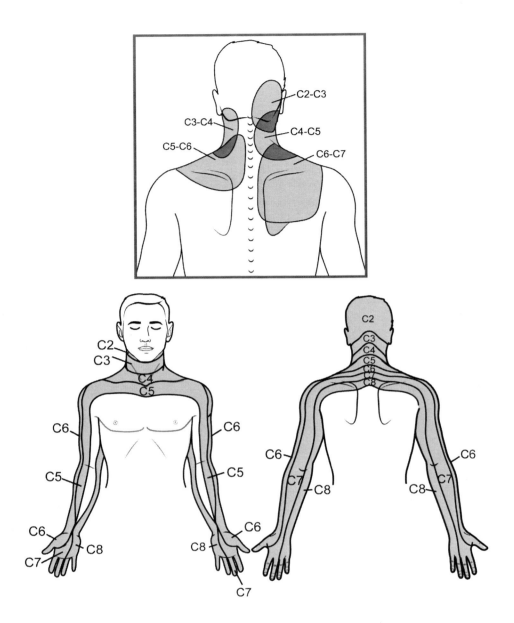

Inflammation of the cervical nerves can create pain in different areas of the shoulder.

gets worse as you turn your head from side to side or look up and down. This happens because these types of neck movements may irritate the already inflamed structure in your cervical spine that is creating the shoulder pain.

The front of the spine in the neck is made up of a disc with a bone called a vertebra on either side of the disc. The back of the spine is held together at each level by a joint called a facet. The nerve exits out of the hole, called the foramen, on the side of the spine. (**Picture 65**).

Picture 66 shows you the different possibilities that can irritate the nerve. This nerve can become inflamed by a bulging or herniated disc pressing on the nerve, or because the foramen has been narrowed by arthritis. So your shoulder can hurt if the C5, C6, or C7 nerve in your cervical spine becomes inflamed, either because of a disc herniation or because the foramen is narrowed.

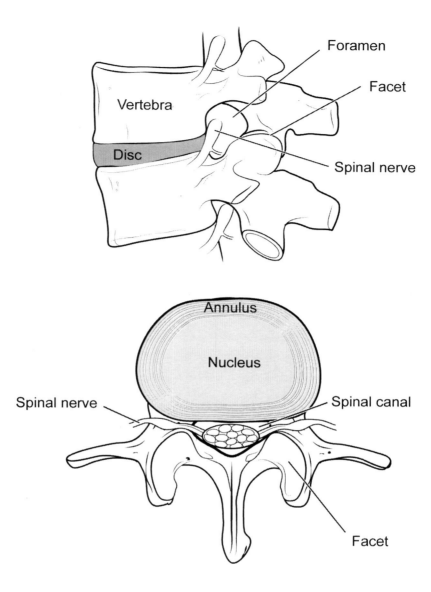

PICTURE 65

The structures of
the spine.

So in summary, the C4-C5, C5-C6, and C6-C7 structures, whether nerve, disc, or facet, can refer pain to the front and/or back of the shoulder **(Picture 67)**.

By now you know that your shoulder pain can be created by an issue with your neck and, of course, by the shoulder itself. So the three common causes of shoulder pain are as follows:

1. Arthritis of the shoulder joint. The wear and tear of arthritis is characterized by progressive wearing away of the cartilage of the joint. It usually creates pain on activity and limits range of motion of the shoulder joint. Patients may feel a grinding or catching within the joint. This type of pain usually does not go down the arm, stays primarily in the front of the shoulder, and rarely creates pain in the area of the shoulder blade. Pain never will go past the elbow.

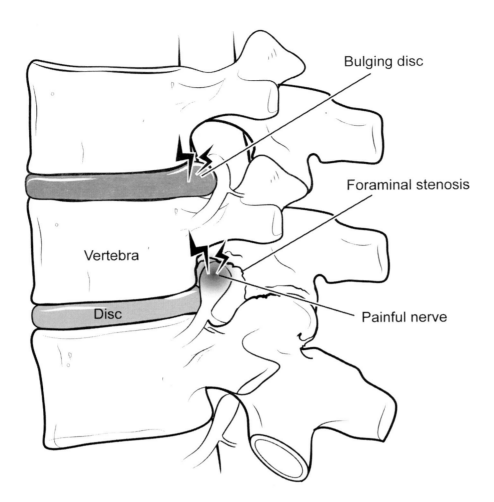

Bulging disc

Foraminal stenosis

Vertebra

Disc

Painful nerve

Inflamed cervical nerve caused by a disc herniation or foraminal stenosis.

2. Bursitis of the shoulder joint. This pain is due to some form of pinching of the tendons and bursa of the rotator cuff between the bones. Often, an initial injury sets off the process of inflammation. Common symptoms include pain with overhead activities and pain while sleeping at night. The pain usually is over the front of the shoulder or the top of the shoulder and upper arm, but it is never past the elbow and never goes down to the shoulder blade.

3. Cervical spine creating shoulder pain. This is the only one of the three common causes of shoulder pain that usually creates pain in the arm below the elbow, as well as in the shoulder blade. Most patients will notice that their pain begins spontaneously and may even occur at night. Patients have told me that they awaken with a "crick" in their neck, and then the pain gets worse over the next several days. You may have shoulder pain that actually is coming from the neck without having any neck pain, and it may mimic bursitis of the shoulder by creating pain with motion of the shoulder. Pain that originates in the neck and runs all the way down the arm most commonly comes from the neck. If an inflamed cervical nerve is creating your shoulder pain, you may feel better if you raise your arm over your shoulder and put it on top of your head because this position takes the pressure off the nerve.

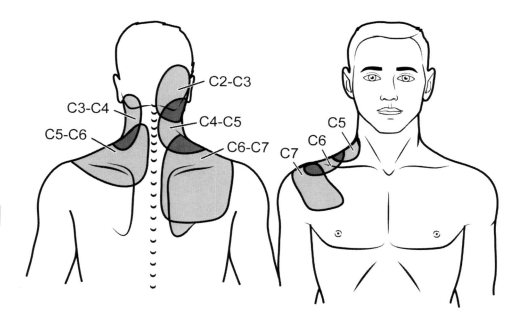

PICTURE 67

Shoulder pain created by inflamed cervical discs, facet joints, and/or nerves.

Why not just get an MRI of the shoulder or of the cervical spine to find the problem? Because the MRI shows degeneration and wear and tear. It does not show pain. One thing you must remember is that you can have all sorts of degeneration in your shoulder and cervical spine yet have *no pain*. A shoulder MRI may show significant wear and tear, yet you may find that the pain is not coming from the shoulder. The same is true for your cervical spine. As we age, all of our discs are going to degenerate and protrude. Most of our facets or joints are going to get arthritic, and the holes where the nerves exit are going to narrow. And most of the time, no pain is associated with these changes. The bottom line is to diagnose the problem *before* you obtain an MRI. Then use the MRI to narrow down the issue. And finally use the minimally invasive diagnostic procedures described in Chapter 16 to find and treat the problem at the same time.

This seemingly complicated issue with trying to determine whether the shoulder pain is coming from the shoulder or the neck can be easily diagnosed with these minimally invasive diagnostic procedures. All your doctor has to do is use an X-ray machine, numb the inside of the shoulder with a local anesthetic, and see whether the shoulder pain is gone. If the pain is gone, you know that the pain probably is coming from the shoulder. If the pain is not gone, you know that your pain may be referred from the neck. Then the minimally invasive diagnostic procedures can locate the exact structure in the neck that is creating the shoulder pain. These same procedures are used therapeutically to eradicate the inflammation to provide long-term relief. And if you do not get long-term relief, you will know the exact problem that needs to be fixed.

SUMMARY

1. Shoulder pain can come from the cervical spine or the shoulder.

2. It is essential to know whether it is your shoulder or one of the structures in your cervical spine (nerve, facet joint, or disc) that is creating the pain.

3. The therapy and treatment for each one is quite different.

4. Read Chapters 2 and 3 to find out more about the structures of the cervical spine and how they create shoulder pain.

5. Chapter 16 will explain how to diagnose shoulder pain with minimally invasive procedures.

6. Chapter 17 provides information about therapy and exercises for shoulder pain.

CHAPTER 9

My Neck Hurts

I see a lot of patients who have neck pain without any discomfort going down the arm or into the shoulder. You may notice that along with your neck pain you have some level of muscle spasm in the neck and even headaches that go up the back of the skull. The pain can be worse in the morning or throughout the day, and the discomfort may be aggravated by looking up, looking down, or turning your head to either side. Most patients tell me that they cannot remember anything specific that started their pain, whereas some say they just noticed a "crick" in their neck, and yet others tell me that it started with a generalized soreness of their neck. The neck pain may get better for a while and then suddenly become severe for absolutely no reason. Let's talk about a pain in the neck.

Each segment of the cervical spine (whether the disc, the nerve, or the facet joint) can create neck pain when inflamed. **Picture 68** illustrates where each segment of the cervical spine creates pain. The C2-C3 segment, when inflamed, creates upper neck pain that goes into the skull, and the C3-C4 segment causes neck pain that starts from the ear and goes to the top of the shoulder. The C4-C5 disc or facet, when inflamed, creates pain from the upper neck to the shoulder. The last two levels in the cervical spine, C5-C6 and C6-C7, create neck pain that also may go down into the shoulder. As you can see, there is some overlap between the segments—so, for example,

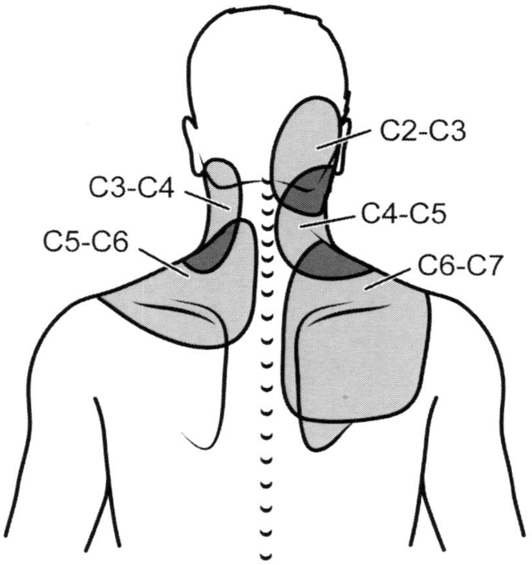

PICTURE 68

Areas of pain resulting from inflammation of a cervical disc, nerve, or facet.

the C5-C6 segment can create pain into the middle of the neck, which is an area also covered by the C4-C5 segment.

Picture 69 shows that each segment in the neck consists of a disc, facet joint, and nerve. Any one of the three structures at the C5-C6 level (disc, facet, or nerve) can create pain in the C5-C6 area of the neck as seen in Picture 68.

You may be thinking that all you need to do to find the problem creating your neck pain is to get an MRI of your cervical spine. Unfortunately, it is not that easy. All an MRI is going to show is wear and tear. It does not show pain.

As we age, all of our discs and joints are going to degenerate: half the world population by age fifty will have disc herniations and arthritic facet joints. And this number only goes up as we get older. By the time we are in our sixties and seventies, most of us are going to have multiple disc herniations and arthritic joints.

The *good news* is that even though a level of wear and tear comes with getting old, most of those changes, whether a large disc herniation or an arthritic joint, will *not* create much pain. You only will have pain when the structures in your neck become inflamed.

The *bad news* is that the MRI does not actually tell you which of the degenerated areas is creating the pain. How do you find the disc herniation, nerve, or arthritic facet joint that is creating the inflammation when you do

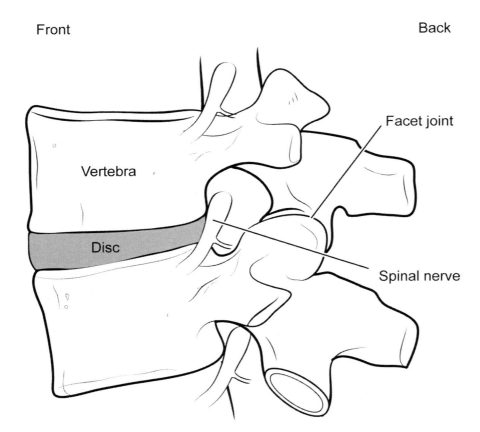

Front

Back

Facet joint

Vertebra

Disc

Spinal nerve

PICTURE 69

Parts of the cervical spine.

hurt, when most disc herniations and arthritic changes that you find on an MRI do not create pain?

You try to pin down the problem *before* you have the MRI, and then see whether the MRI matches up to your area of pain. By using the following method, the therapeutic results are much better. I ask the patients first to fill out a pain diagram that shows the specific area where the patient feels pain. Let me give you several examples.

Picture 70 shows that the patient's pain is located in the neck with the pain going up toward the bottom of the skull and wrapping around to the area of the ear. If you match that information with Picture 68, you now know that this patient's pain probably is coming from the C2-C3 or C3-C4 segment. Identifying the specific area where you are feeling pain will give you a head start in locating the painful structure. If I obtain an MRI and see disc herniations at C3-C4 and C6-C7, I would then use a minimally invasive procedure to see if the C3-C4 disc is the possible cause of the pain.

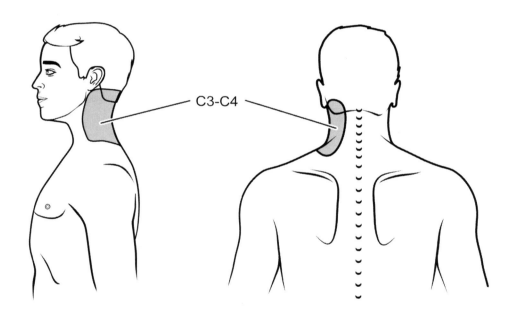

PICTURE 70

Area of pain caused by inflammation at the C3-C4 level.

Picture 71 shows an example of a patient with neck pain going down into the shoulder. If you compare Picture 71 with Picture 68, you notice that it appears to match the C4-C5 or C5-C6 area. It does not tell you whether the joint, the disc, or the nerve is creating the pain, but it gives you a general area to start. Remember, some segments overlap, so you may have an issue with C4-C5 or C5-C6, but we are narrowing down the problem. The next step is to find which of the three structures at that level (the disc, the facet joint, or the nerve) is creating your pain. Let me give you some information about these different structures.

When cervical discs are inflamed, they will create pain in the areas shown in Picture 68 depending on the level. So an inflamed C2-C3 disc will give you pain

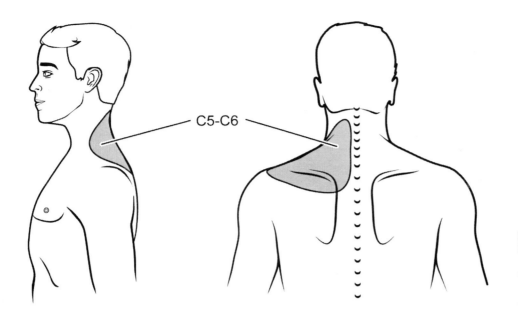

PICTURE 71

Area of pain caused by inflammation at the C5-C6 level.

at the bottom of your skull, whereas the C6-C7 will create pain in the neck going down to the shoulder blade. You may notice that your pain comes and goes and that on some days it is terrible and on other days quite mild. Patients with disc pain usually feel okay when they first get up in the morning, but the pain gets worse throughout the day because the weight of the head and gravity create pressure on the disc. Driving in a car or sitting at a desk with your head down are common times when you will note pain. The disc is in the front of your spine, and, as **Picture 72** shows, bending your head forward will increase the pressure on the disc. Patients with inflamed discs do not like looking down for long periods of time because it creates pain.

Rotating your head also creates stress on the disc, as does bending your head sideways. If one of your cervical discs is inflamed, any of these

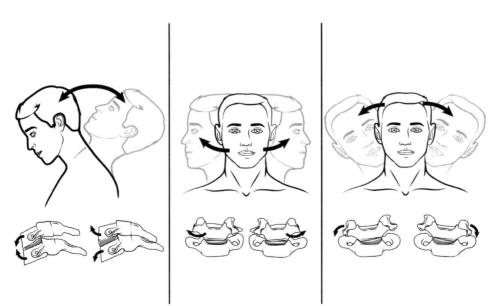

PICTURE 72

Bending the head down or twisting and turning the neck increases stress on the discs.

movements may increase your pain. This is why I am always bugging patients to turn their whole body instead of just their necks and to keep their head up when they are reading or working on a computer!

The facet, or joint, is in the back of the spine (**Picture 73**). The facet joint opens when you bend your neck forward, as when you look down, and has more pressure placed on it when you arch your head backward.

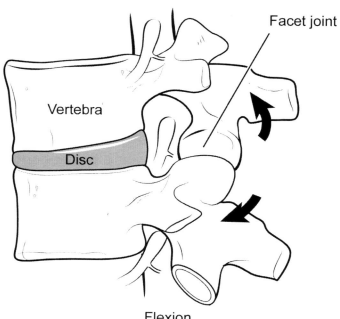

Facet joint

Vertebra

Disc

Flexion
(bending the head forward)

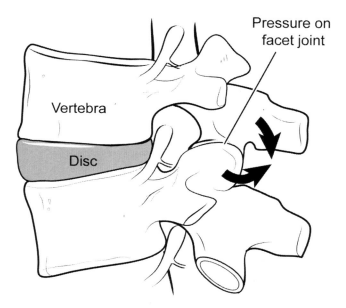

Pressure on
facet joint

Vertebra

Disc

Extension
(bending the head backward)

PICTURE 73

Facet joints open when you bend your head forward and press on each other when you bend your head backward.

Inflamed facet joints create pain primarily in the neck and shoulders, but the pain never goes down the arm. The pain usually is worse when you get up in the morning, especially if you are lying on your back or stomach, as the joints have been pressing on each other all night because of the position of your neck. If your facets are inflamed, you usually will notice that your neck hurts when you look up or turn your head, as those motions can aggravate the joints and create pain. Patients with inflamed facet joint pain in the neck try to keep the head down so that the joints stay open. You may also notice popping sounds as you turn or twist your neck. Picture 68 shows where each of the joints creates pain in the neck and shoulders.

The cervical nerves exit the holes, or foramen, on the side of the spine and then go to different areas of the neck, shoulder, and arm (**Picture 74**). The nerve can become inflamed either because of a disc herniation irritating it or because of the narrowing of the hole where the nerve exits, which is called foraminal stenosis.

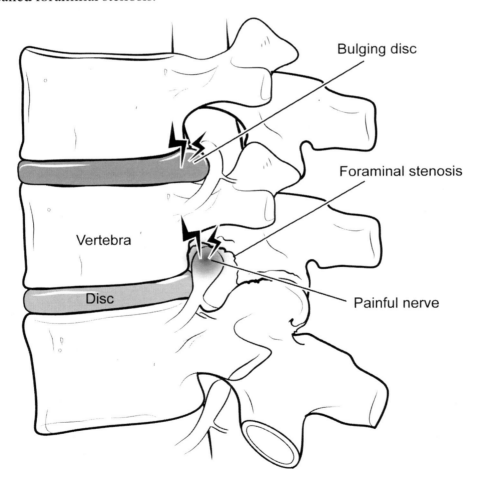

Bulging disc

Foraminal stenosis

Vertebra

Disc

Painful nerve

PICTURE 74

Inflamed painful nerve because of a bulging disc or foraminal stenosis.

As you can see in **Picture 75**, every one of the cervical nerves covers some part of the neck, even the ones that continue down the arm. The cervical nerves C5, C6, and C7 and the first thoracic nerve T1 all go down the arm, but first they go to the neck and shoulders.

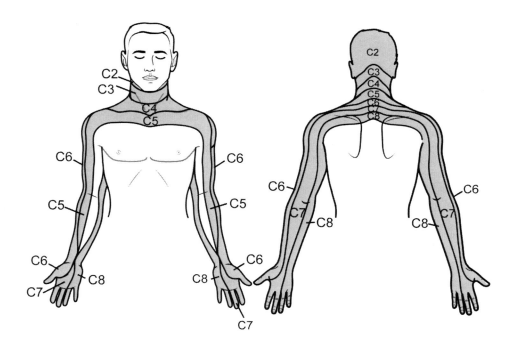

PICTURE 75

The areas of the body where you will feel pain when each specific cervical nerve is inflamed.

You do not have to have pain going down the arm or shoulder every time a cervical nerve is inflamed. The pain you feel may only be in the neck. **Picture 76** shows where each one of the cervical nerves can create pain in the neck and shoulder without actually going down the arms.

A lot of patients have been told that because their pain is not going down the arm, it must not be caused by the nerve. After treating a lot of patients, I have found that the most likely cause of any pain in the neck, shoulder, or arm is one of the nerves in the cervical spine, not the disc or the facet. You have to find the exact structure that is creating your neck pain if you want it

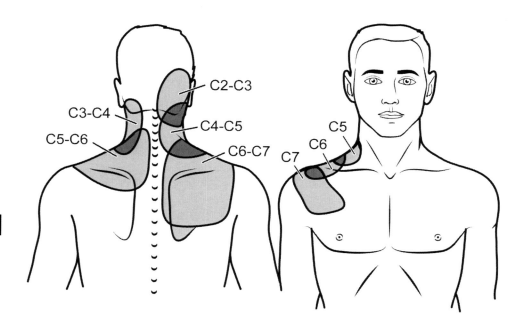

PICTURE 76

Neck and shoulder pain created by the cervical nerves when they are inflamed.

to go away. I am going to discuss the specifics of how I go about diagnosing the exact nerve, facet, or disc that is creating your neck pain in Chapter 16.

One type of neck pain worth noting is upper neck pain that goes up the back of the skull. Patients with this type of pain may have been diagnosed with migraines or "occipital neuralgia," which is an inflammation of the nerves that go up the back of the skull. These patients at times have actually had an inflamed disc, nerve, or joint in their cervical spine creating their headaches or upper neck pain. **Picture 77** shows that the disc between C2-C3, the nerve from C2 or C3, or the facet joints from the C1-C2 or C2-C3 levels can create pain in the upper neck and in the back of the skull and head. I have also found that when any of the discs, joints, or nerves in the neck are inflamed, they can create muscle spasms in the neck and, in turn, cause headaches. Therefore, even a C6-C7 disc or a C4-C5 facet may create headaches. Once the inflammation in the specific structure is eradicated, the headaches usually subside.

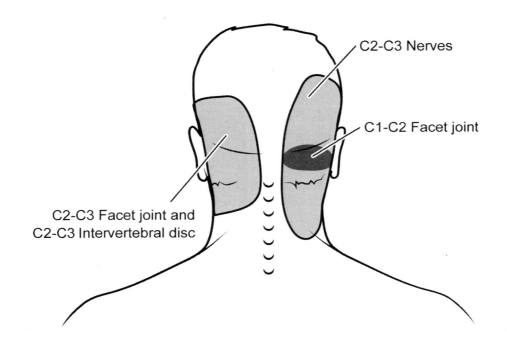

C2-C3 Nerves

C1-C2 Facet joint

C2-C3 Facet joint and
C2-C3 Intervertebral disc

PICTURE 77

Pain in the upper neck, skull, and back of the head can be due to structures in the spine.

SUMMARY

1. Neck pain is usually created by the inflammation of one of the structures in the cervical spine, whether it is the disc, the facet joint, or the nerve.

2. It is important to locate the exact structure in the cervical spine that is creating the problem if you want pain relief.

3. Chapters 2 and 3 provide more information regarding the cervical structures that create neck pain.

4. Chapter 16 discusses the diagnostic and therapeutic approach to this type of neck pain.

5. Chapter 17 provides information on therapy and exercises for your neck.

My Arm Hurts—It Tingles and My Fingers Go Numb

Multiple medical problems other than an issue with the cervical spine can create arm pain. These problems include an entrapment or compression of the nerves after they leave the neck, such as carpal tunnel syndrome or thoracic outlet syndrome. Also, problems with muscles or bones in the arm may create discomfort. I am going to focus on the problems with the nerves in the cervical spine that can create arm pain.

In Chapters 8 and 9, I talked about how the cervical nerves can create shoulder and neck pain. These same nerves in the neck can create arm pain. If you look at **Picture 78**, you will see that the nerves starting at C5 and going down to C8 can all create pain in some part of the arm. The C8 nerve travels down the inside of the arm to the back part of the elbow, also called the funny bone, and then continues to the little finger. The C7 nerve goes down the back of the arm to the elbow and then goes to the hand and middle fingers. The C6 nerve descends more on the outside of the arm to the front of the elbow, goes through the forearm and then to the thumb and first finger. The C5 nerve goes down the front and top of the shoulder and then down the front of the arm to the forearm.

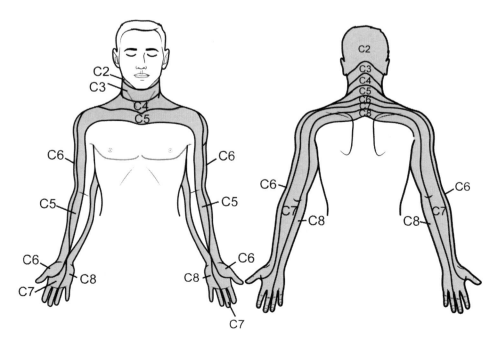

PICTURE 78

Areas of the body that will be painful depending on which cervical nerve is inflamed.

One of the most common symptoms of neck and arm pain due to the cervical spine is that the pain may not be continuous. The arm pain can be terrible at times, and then it can get a lot better for a while or even disappear completely. Nerve pain usually is worse at night as the position of lying down, which most of us think should be restful, at times can create a mechanical irritation of the nerve. On several occasions, I have had to sleep in an upright position just to be able to rest. The inflamed nerve feels better when tension on the nerve is reduced, and therefore patients may keep their arm raised over their head to give the nerve some slack.

Certain positions of your neck can make arm pain better or worse. Turning your head toward the side that hurts usually makes the pain worse because it can create an irritation of the nerve, and turning your head to the side opposite your pain may feel better as it gives the disc and the nerve room to breathe. Looking down may increase the pain as that position may create more pressure on your disc and nerve, and you might notice that you tend to arch your neck because that will take the pressure off the disc. But depending on the position of the disc herniation, at other times your pain will get worse when you arch your neck and you may feel better looking down. When you are in a lot of pain, you are going to hold your head, neck, and arm in whatever position gives you relief. And that is the correct position. You cannot fight pain over posture. Let the body hold itself in whatever position it needs to give it pain relief, and try not to worry about posture while you are in pain.

The C5, C6, and C7 nerves may create pain only in the arm, but usually they will create pain into the front and back of the shoulder at the same time. **Picture 79** shows where each of these nerves may create pain in the neck and shoulder area. The nerves also can create pain just in the neck and shoulder area without going down the arms.

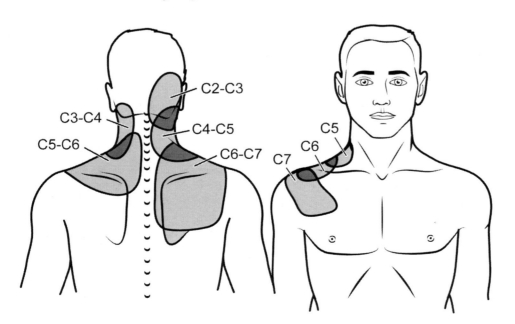

PICTURE 79

The C5, C6, and C7 nerves can create pain in the shoulder without going down the arm.

So far I have discussed arm pain, but you also can have numbness, tingling, and even weakness at times. Each nerve is made up of different components, including fibers that carry pain signals, create sensation in the arm, and give the muscles strength. These fibers, when inflamed or irritated, can create pain, numbness, and weakness. At times, you may notice symptoms of any combination of these three. So, for example, the C6 nerve when inflamed can create pain down the shoulder and arm, along with numbness and tingling into the fingers, especially the thumb and first finger (**Picture 80**).

The C7 nerve when inflamed can create pain in the back of your arm, knife-like pain in the back of the shoulder, and numbness and tingling in your middle three fingers (**Picture 81**).

The great news for these types of pain is that they usually are self-limiting. Within four to six weeks, most of the symptoms will be gone. This is usually true no matter what type of conservative care you undergo—whether the pain is managed by medications, physical therapy, or just putting up with the discomfort. During this period of time, you just need to find a way to make the pain tolerable and wait for the body to take care of the situation. It will be time to move to the next step if the pain does not clear in four to six weeks. An MRI of the neck can be used to verify what we already know by

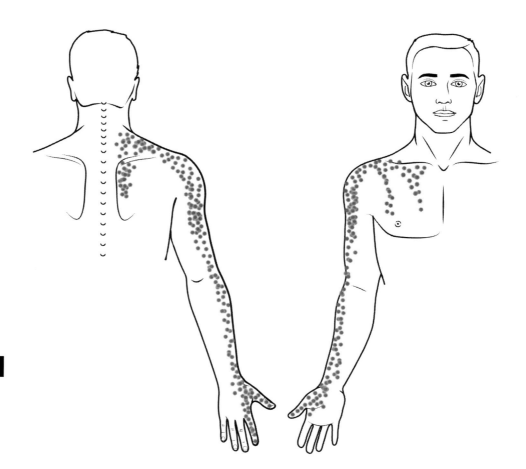

PICTURE 80

The areas of the body that will be painful when the C6 nerve is inflamed.

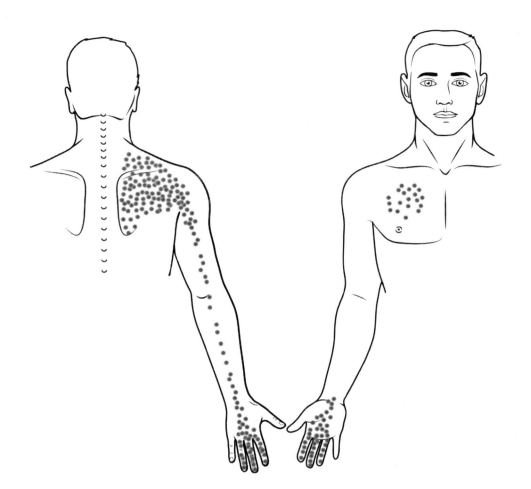

PICTURE 81

The areas of the body that will be painful when the C7 nerve is inflamed.

the history and clinical exam. Then, by using the minimally invasive diagnostic procedures detailed in Chapter 16, you can locate the exact nerve that is creating your pain and treat it therapeutically at the same time.

Remember, other things can create pain in the arm. Carpal tunnel syndrome, which compresses the nerve in the wrist area and creates numbness and pain in the hand, or cubital tunnel syndrome, which creates a compression of a nerve in the area of the elbow and numbness and pain in the little finger, are two common problems that also can cause pain, numbness, or weakness in the arm. It is important to ensure that you know exactly what is creating your symptoms *before* treating the problem.

SUMMARY

1. The cervical nerves C5, C6, C7, and C8 can create pain, numbness, and weakness in your arm when they are inflamed. Each nerve covers a specific area of the arm, and they usually create pain in the neck or shoulder at the same time.

2. Cervical nerve pain usually resolves itself within several weeks. During this time, medications, physical therapy, and being careful not to aggravate your neck are all that you need.

3. If the pain continues past that time, then obtain an MRI and consider a minimally invasive diagnostic procedure. This will allow you to locate the exact nerve that is creating your pain as well as therapeutically treating it at the same time.

4. Chapters 2 and 3 provide more information on the cervical nerves.

5. Chapter 16 will give you diagnostic and treatment options.

6. Chapter 17 provides information about therapy if you are hurting and exercises once your pain has resolved.

My Mid-Back Hurts—I Feel Like I Pulled a Muscle

The level of the spine that creates pain in the mid-back area is called the thoracic spine, which is between the cervical and lumbar segments. Like the cervical and lumbar spine, the thoracic spine has discs, joints, and nerves. This is the longest area of the spine, with twelve vertebrae compared with seven for the cervical and five for the lumbar (**Picture 82**). The thoracic spine causes fewer episodes of pain than the cervical (neck) and lumbar (lower back) segments of the spine. The reason is that most of the bending and twisting of the human spine takes place in the cervical and lumbar areas. Also, ribs are attached to each of the thoracic vertebrae, providing additional support to the thoracic spine and therefore decreasing the amount of movement in this part of the spine.

I used to think that the thoracic area of the spine created minimal pain because there is not as much movement in this segment of the spine. As the years have gone by, however, I continue to see a lot of patients with undiagnosed pain from this area of the spine. They most commonly complain about pain in the area of their shoulder blade, a pulled muscle in the middle of the back, pain wrapping into the front of their chest, or even discomfort that they thought was from a hernia or some other abdominal problem as the pain may wrap into the groin or abdominal area. Again, I caution you that not all pain in this area is from the spine, *but* if you continue to hurt in these areas and everything else has been ruled out, you should keep this chapter in mind.

The reason the thoracic spine is unique is that each thoracic nerve, after it exits the hole or foramen, is attached to the bottom of a rib. **Picture 83** shows that the nerves in this area of the body wrap around the mid-back and travel all the way to the front of the body.

When the thoracic nerve that wraps around the rib becomes inflamed, you may notice muscle spasms and pain in any of the areas covered by these nerves. You may notice pain in your mid-back, the side of your rib, or even the front of your body, all due to the same nerve.

Picture 84 illustrates where the different nerves run in the thoracic spine. The nerves start in the mid-back and wrap around to the chest, abdomen, hip, and groin. Remember, you may feel pain in any area along the path of these nerves.

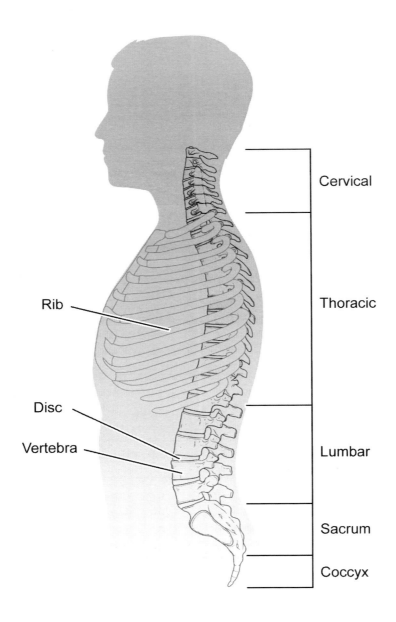

Cervical

Thoracic

Rib

Disc

Vertebra

Lumbar

Sacrum

Coccyx

PICTURE 82

The thoracic spine with attachment of ribs.

These nerves most commonly become inflamed because of a disc herniation pushing against the nerve or because the hole from which the nerve exits is narrowed and creates nerve irritation. You may notice that the pain is isolated in the middle of your back, or you may feel that the pain starts on one side of your mid-back and wraps around your chest or abdomen. Some patients feel a "catch" under their ribs, or they think their rib is broken even though they have not had any trauma to that part of the body.

The pain may get worse with specific movements that place pressure on the disc, which in turn can aggravate the pain from the nerve. Bending forward and twisting motions are two common movements that can aggravate this type of pain. Patients will notice that sitting for an extended period of time can make the pain worse because this puts a lot of pressure on the discs (**Picture 85**).

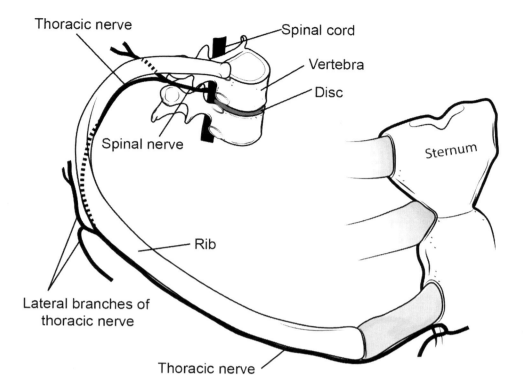

Thoracic nerve

Spinal cord

Vertebra

Disc

Sternum

Spinal nerve

Rib

Lateral branches of
thoracic nerve

Thoracic nerve

PICTURE 83

The thoracic nerve
starts in the back of
the body and wraps all
the way around to the
front of the abdomen
and chest.

We tend to sit slumped over in our chairs, a position that increases pressure on the disc, which, over a period of time, may inflame the nerve. To avoid this problem, you need to sit in a correct position with your spine held straight and make it a point to get up and walk around every hour so that the disc will not have constant pressure on it. Even better, stand up while working. The best position for the spine usually is standing as it takes the pressure off the discs compared with the sitting position. I have converted most of my own workplaces to sit-stand desks that can move up and down. I also stress the importance of using your legs to do most of the bending to reduce pressure on the disc. When you bend over without bending your knees, you increase the pressure inside the disc. This increased pressure, in turn, can either aggravate the nerve or create inflammation inside the disc.

An MRI of the mid-back or thoracic area may *not* show an obvious herniation or narrowing of the hole from which the nerve exits, even though you are in pain. I have seen countless patients who have *not* been treated because of the lack of findings on the MRI. The MRI is done with the patient lying down, and therefore the changes that occur when the weight of the body is on the disc may be missed. The MRI may not show the true clinical picture, as it may miss the inflammation inside the disc. The MRI is not the diagnostic tool that everyone thinks it is. I always go by the history and clinical picture and use the MRI as a secondary tool.

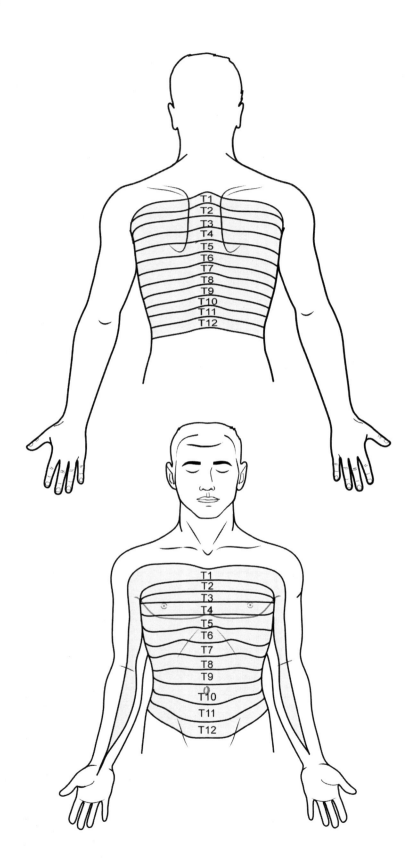

PICTURE 84

The areas of the body that are painful when specific thoracic nerves are inflamed.

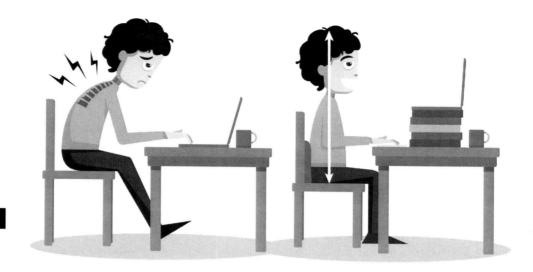

PICTURE 85

Proper posture when you sit at a computer.

One area of the mid-back that seems to cause confusion is pain in the shoulder blade. This area of pain can be coming from the thoracic spine or can be referred from the cervical spine. First look at Picture 84 and see what level of the thoracic nerves covers the shoulder blade. You will notice that it can be any of the nerves from T3 to T7. Now look at **Picture 86**. Here you can see that the pain in the shoulder blade area usually is covered by any of the cervical nerves from C5 through C7. This area of pain coincides with that caused by the T3 to T7 nerves.

So is your pain coming from the thoracic or the cervical spine? An easy way to diagnose this is by running a pinwheel or a paper clip down that area of the spine. If you detect an area of hypersensitivity as you drag the pinwheel or paper clip down past the area of pain, the pain is usually coming

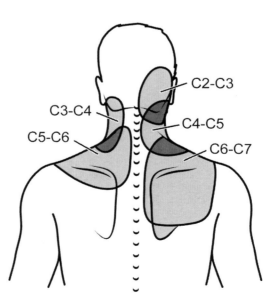

PICTURE 86

The areas of the shoulder that will hurt when specific cervical nerves are inflamed.

from a nerve in the thoracic spine. If there is no hypersensitivity, then the pain possibly is being referred from the cervical spine. Other symptoms may also help determine which part of the spine is creating the pain. If it is coming from the cervical spine, you may have neck or arm pain as well as shoulder blade pain. You may notice that the shoulder blade pain increases if you turn your neck or look up or down. If the pain is coming from the thoracic spine, you will not have any symptoms in the neck or arm. An MRI may help determine where your pain originates if it shows a disc herniation or arthritis in the same area as your discomfort. Once I have collected all this information, I use minimally invasive diagnostic procedures to determine the exact nerve or disc that is creating the pain. The diagnosis and treatment of the thoracic nerve and disc are addressed in Chapter 16.

The last structures that can create pain in the thoracic spine are the facet joints that are located in the back of the spine. I find the facet joints to be an unusual cause of pain in the thoracic area, as most of the discomfort in the thoracic area is due to the disc or nerve. As you can see in **Picture 87**, the thoracic facets open up when you bend your thoracic spine forward, and the joints press on each other when you bend backward.

If the thoracic facets are inflamed you will notice that your pain gets worse when you bend backward or arch your back (extension) and feels better when you bend forward. This is the opposite of disc pain, which gets worse when you bend forward (flexion) and feels better when you arch your back. Facet pain does not wrap around the ribs to the side or front of your body. The pain from these joints is usually worse when you first wake up, if you sleep on your back. Patients with facet pain will feel better by lying on their side in a fetal position as that position keeps the facet joint open.

One more structure that should be mentioned is the vertebra itself. In people over the age of fifty, especially when these patients have osteoporosis, the thoracic vertebrae have a tendency to fracture and create significant acute pain in the mid-back area. These are called vertebral compression fractures (**Picture 88**).

The patient with a vertebral compression fracture may have sudden, severe back pain, or it may come on gradually over time. The fracture may start as a mild back strain when the patient does something like bend forward or twist. It may be the result of a common activity like bending over to pick something up or lifting a bag of groceries.

The pain from a compression fracture is worse when standing or walking, and it gets better when the patient sits down or lies down and does not move. The pain usually feels worse when the patient bends or twists. The fracture can irritate the thoracic nerve that runs at the same level as the fracture and can create pain that wraps around to the front of the chest. This type of pain can be treated conservatively if the patient wears a brace and

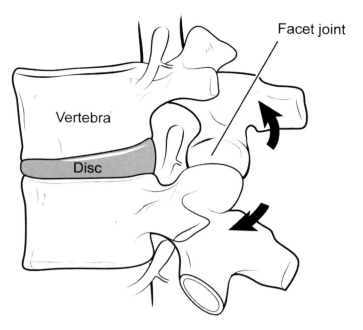

Flexion (bending forward)

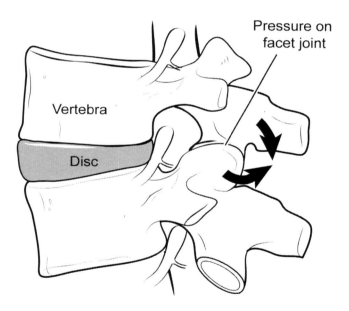

Extension
(arching the back or bending backward)

PICTURE 87

Thoracic facet joints open when you bend forward and press on each other when you bend backward.

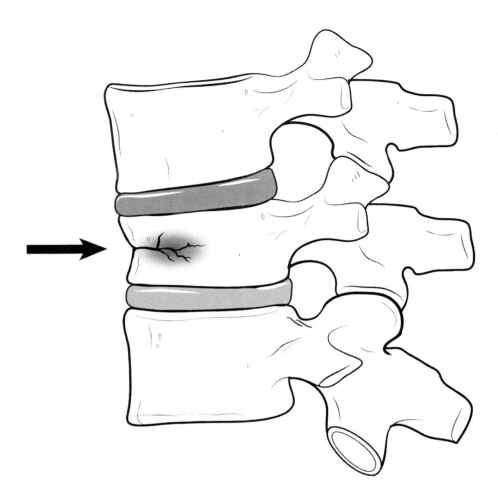

Vertebral compression fracture.

takes oral pain medications. Most fractures will heal over several weeks. If the pain is severe or continues after several weeks, a course of steroids can be administered in the area of the nerve to eradicate the inflammation. If needed, cement can be placed in the fracture to fix it. I advocate doing this only as a last resort, because cementing the fracture places significant stress on the vertebrae above and below the fracture and subsequently makes these vertebrae prone to fractures.

SUMMARY

1. Thoracic pain, which is pain in the area of the mid-back, is a lot more common than most medical practitioners realize.

2. The thoracic discs, nerves, and facet joints can create pain in the area of the ribs, shoulder blade, upper back, chest, abdomen, and groin in addition to the middle of the back.

3. For more detailed information about the thoracic spine, read Chapters 2 and 3.

4. The diagnosis and treatment of thoracic pain are reviewed in Chapter 16.

5. Chapter 17 teaches you exercises to strengthen the thoracic area of your spine.

CHAPTER 12

My Pain Is in My Buttock

Pain in the buttock area is one of the most common reasons why patients come to see me. All the diagnoses that I discuss in this chapter explain why you might have pain in the buttock area, but the number one problem that I have seen that creates buttock pain is an inflammation of one of the structures of the lumbar spine.

I am not saying that buttock pain cannot be caused by an inflammation of the hip, sacroiliac joint, piriformis muscle, or hamstring muscle. But these causes are way down the list. Most of the time you will find that one of the nerves in the lumbar or sacral spine is inflamed, and therefore it creates pain that goes into your buttock. **Picture 89** shows the areas of the *skin* over the buttocks that these nerves go to once the nerves come out of your lumbar spine. This is usually the picture that most medical practitioners look at. As you can see in Picture 89, the L5, S1, S2, and S3 lumbar and sacral nerves cover the surface of the buttock area. If one of these nerves is inflamed, it can create pain anywhere along the path of the nerve. So you can have buttock pain from the L5 nerve *without* having any leg pain or back pain. One of the most common reasons why medical practitioners start thinking about other diagnoses for buttock pain is that they expect the lumbar nerves to always create back and leg pain at the same time the patient is having buttock pain.

The next picture is not one that is commonly considered by medical practitioners but is very important when it comes to buttock pain. **Picture 90** shows you where the lumbar nerves go to the *muscles* and *bones* of the buttock area. If you look at the right-hand image, you will see that the lumbar nerves L3, L4, and L5 as well as the S1 nerve can create pain in the *muscles* and *bones* of the buttock. In the right-hand image, the lower buttock area is covered by the L3 and L4 nerves. These nerves are not commonly considered to create pain in the buttock area, but I have seen many patients who have buttock pain because the lumbar nerves at the L3 and L4 levels are inflamed. So between these last two pictures you can now see how almost any lumbar and sacral nerve can create buttock pain!

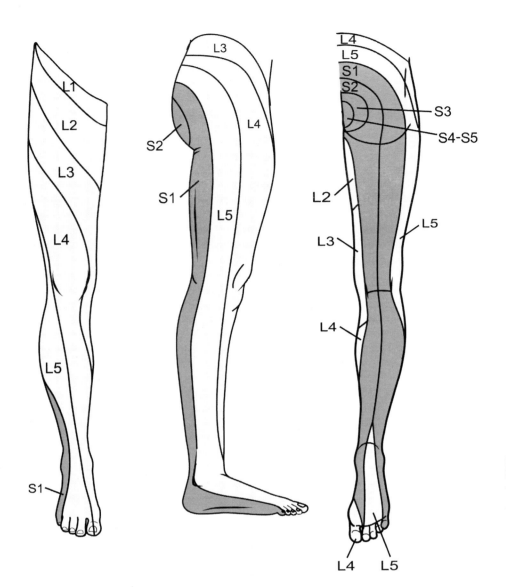

PICTURE 89

The areas of the body that will be painful depending on which specific lumbar nerve is inflamed.

Front of body

Back of body

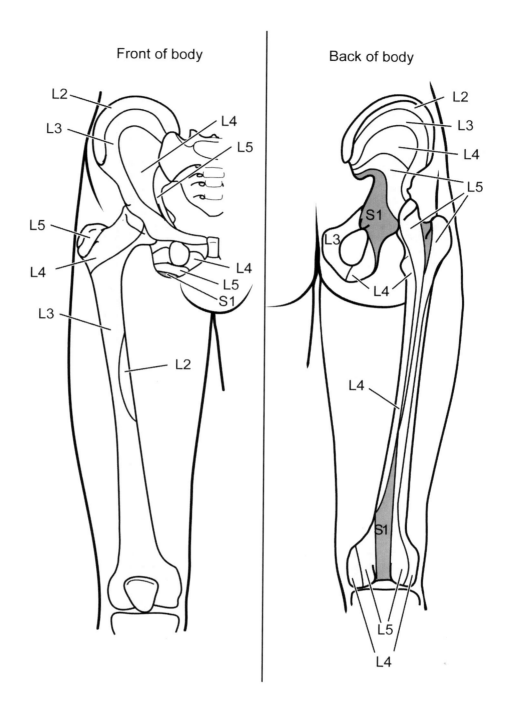

PICTURE 90

Areas of the buttock, groin, and hip that will hurt depending on which lumbar nerve is inflamed.

Some of these same patients have been told that their pain was coming from their piriformis muscle or their sacroiliac joint because they had pain in those areas. The nerves in the lumbar spine go to all of the muscles and bones in the buttock area, including the piriformis muscle and the sacroiliac joint, and therefore when these nerves are inflamed in the spine, these muscles and joints can be quite painful. But these muscles and joints are painful because of your problem in your lumbar spine, *not* because there is anything wrong with your piriformis muscle or sacroiliac joint. Treat the inflamed lumbar nerve and the pain in the area of the piriformis muscle and sacroiliac joint will go away. Chapter 16 will give you information about how I use minimally invasive techniques to do that.

> **Remember: Most buttock pain is due to an inflammation of one of the nerves in your lumbar spine.**

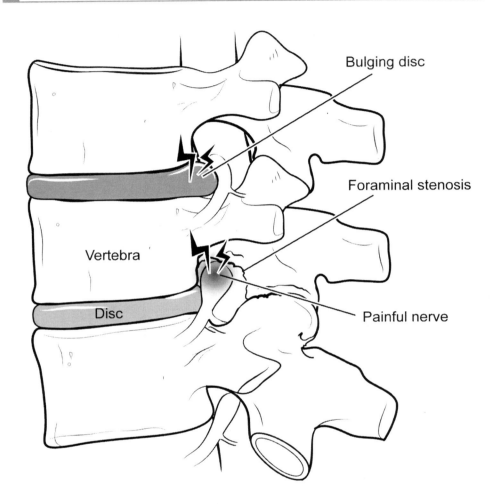

Bulging disc

Foraminal stenosis

Vertebra

Disc

Painful nerve

PICTURE 91

Inflammation of the lumbar nerve due to foraminal stenosis and/or bulging disc.

Two of the most common reasons for a lumbar nerve to become inflamed are a herniated disc irritating the nerve or a narrowing of the hole from which the nerve exits, causing the nerve to become inflamed. The narrowing of the hole, called foraminal stenosis (**Picture 91**), is usually due to arthritic changes in the bone or an enlarged facet joint. Remember, you can have nerve pain originating from the lumbar spine which creates pain in the area of the buttock, but have *no* back or leg pain.

Buttock pain from a disc herniation inflaming the nerve on the side of your spine as the nerve exits, or because the hole is narrowed, is usually worse when you sit, and it feels better when you get up and walk. You can try to sit on the other buttock, the one that does not hurt, and straighten out the leg on the same side as the buttock pain, or you may stand up and walk around to feel better. This provides relief because it takes the pressure off the inflamed nerve.

Two things occur when you are in a sitting position. First, you increase the pressure on your disc because of your body weight, and the nerve may stretch and bend a little while you are in the sitting position (**Picture 92**). Just imagine that the line in the picture going down the leg is the nerve. When you are standing, the nerve is relaxed and at its shortest length. When you sit down, the nerve becomes stretched and bent to accommodate the position of sitting. As long as there is no inflammation, there will be no consequences for this change in the length of the nerve and the increased pressure on the disc. But if the nerve is inflamed, the sitting position will increase the stretch and pressure on the nerve and increase your pain. You will be able to relieve the discomfort by taking the stretch off the nerve, either by straightening the leg or by standing up.

Spinal stenosis is another common reason why you may have buttock pain. Spinal stenosis is a narrowing of the *center* of the spinal canal, due to either a disc herniation or enlarged facet joints or ligaments, which leave less

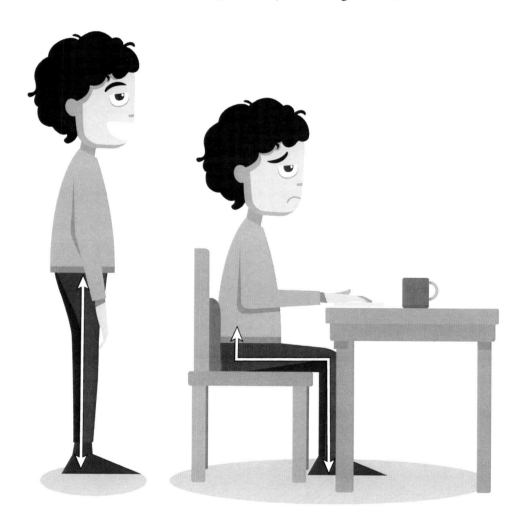

PICTURE 92

Stretching of the nerve when you move to a sitting position.

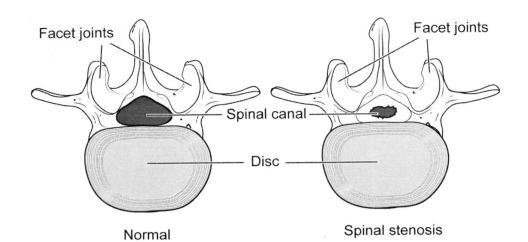

Normal   Spinal stenosis

PICTURE 93

Spinal stenosis.

room for the nerves that go from the lumbar spine into your back, buttocks, and legs **(Picture 93)**. Spinal stenosis usually creates pain in your buttock area when walking or standing, but it gets better with sitting. When you stand or walk, your central canal narrows due to the straightened position of your spine. If you have spinal stenosis because of the limited space in the central canal, the nerves can become inflamed and create pain when you stand or walk. When you sit down, the pain is significantly reduced. These inflamed nerves from the lumbar spine will create pain radiating into the buttock. For more information about spinal stenosis, read Chapter 6.

The joints in the back of the spine, known as the facets, also can create buttock pain **(Picture 94)**. The facet joints open up when you bend forward and close on top of each other when you bend backward, or arch your back. This usually does not create any problems unless your facet joints are inflamed, at which time there may be significant buttock pain, especially when you do things that create pressure on the facet joints, like arching your back or bending backward.

Picture 95 shows where different lumbar facet joints create pain in the buttocks.

One of the worst times for people with inflamed facet joints is in the morning when they first get out of bed, because lying flat in bed creates pressure on these joints. You will usually feel better if you sleep on your side, as that position will put less pressure on your facet joints. When you sit, you will notice that you will feel much better if you sit bent forward to open up your facets. A lumbar support will actually make your pain worse because your spine will be in an arched position. Standing in one place can create pain from inflamed facet joints, which usually is relieved by walking around, because that prevents the facet joints from pressing on each other. Anything to keep your spine from being straight or arched will provide relief.

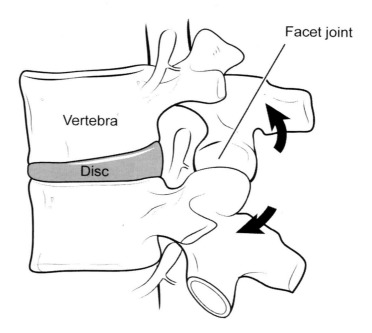

Flexion (bending forward)

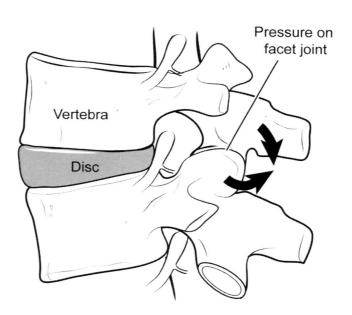

Extension
(arching the back or bending backward)

Facet joints open
when you bend
forward and press on
each other when you
bend backward.

Inflammation of the inside of the disc can create pain that radiates into the buttock. The L4-L5 and the L5-S1 discs usually are the ones that create buttock pain. This pain is usually worse with sitting, as the weight of the body, as well as gravity, creates a lot of pressure on the discs. Patients with disc pain usually squirm in their chairs if they have been sitting for a long time, and they will prefer to stand or walk around. Bending forward increases

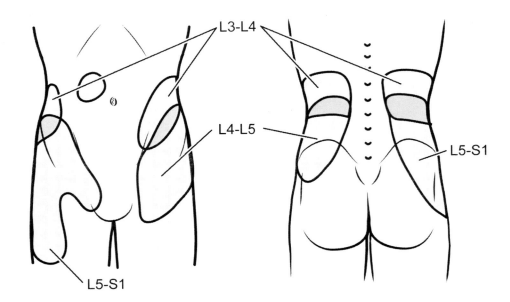

L3-L4

L4-L5

L5-S1

L5-S1

PICTURE 95

The different areas where lumbar facets create pain when they are inflamed.

the pressure in the disc because the discs are in the front of the spine, and if inflamed, they will create pain that may be referred into the buttocks. Patients with disc pain may notice themselves arching their backs at times, as that will relieve the pressure on the disc. This is the exact opposite of patients with facet pain who always are slumped over to keep their facets open.

If the spine has been ruled out, it's time to look at other causes of buttock pain. In no specific order, the following problems can create pain in the buttock area: inflammation of the sacroiliac joint or piriformis muscle, strains or tears of the hamstring muscle, and hip arthritis. This is not a complete list of everything that creates buttock pain, just the most common things that I have seen over the last twenty years.

The sacroiliac joint, which connects the spine and the pelvic bones together, can become inflamed and create buttock pain (**Picture 96**). The sacroiliac joint, found at the lower end of the spine, just below the lumbar spine, is a joint formed between the sacrum and the iliac bone, which is part of the pelvis. This is a large joint that has little motion and involves a limited amount of tilting, sliding, and rotation. The primary function of this joint appears to be to act as a shock absorber and to provide some flexibility to decrease stress on the spine.

The sacroiliac joint commonly is blamed for buttock area pain, but it rarely is the cause. If you look at Pictures 89 and 90, you will see that most of the lumbar nerves cover all of the buttock muscle as well as the bones that make up the sacroiliac joint. Therefore, when any of your lumbar nerves become inflamed, the area around your sacroiliac joint is going to become tender and painful—but not because anything is wrong with your sacroiliac joint. If you treat the lumbar nerve that is inflamed, the pain over your sacroiliac joint will resolve.

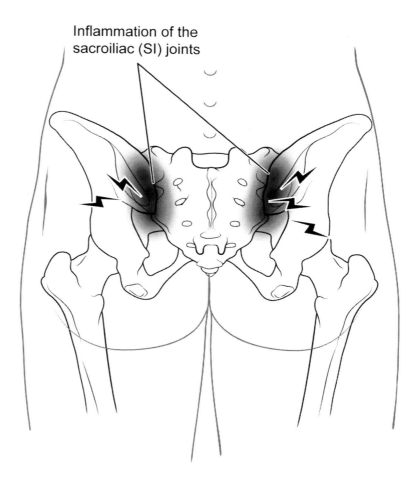

Inflammation of the
sacroiliac (SI) joints

PICTURE 96

Inflammation of the
sacroiliac joint can
create buttock pain.

There are times, however, when the sacroiliac joint does create the buttock pain. Some groups of patients are prone to having sacroiliac joint problems. These include post-pregnancy patients, as pregnancy creates a relaxation of this joint, which therefore becomes more prone to inflammation. Patients with certain forms of arthritis, such as rheumatoid arthritis, psoriasis, and gout also can have an inflamed sacroiliac joint. Some patients have an alignment problem in the spine, which creates stress in this joint and subsequent pain—for example, someone who has had a fusion of the lower part of the spine or scoliosis. The pain from this joint primarily is located in the buttock but also in the groin. The joint may refer pain that goes down the back of the leg but never past the knee.

The most accurate way to decide whether the sacroiliac joint is creating discomfort is to do a diagnostic block of the sacroiliac joint. This can only be done using X-ray guidance because this joint is very small and is deep in the buttock muscle. An anesthetic is injected to numb the sacroiliac joint, and if the pain is gone immediately after the injection, then you can make the diagnosis of sacroiliac joint pain. There is no other way to definitely diagnose this condition, and this procedure cannot be done in an office setting without an X-ray machine, because there is no other way to ensure that the local anesthetic and steroid actually get into the joint. Chapter 16 reviews these diagnostic injections. But remember, the sacroiliac joint pain is *not* a common cause of buttock pain.

The piriformis syndrome is a condition in which the piriformis muscle, which is located in the buttock area, spasms and creates buttock pain (**Picture 97**). The muscle attaches to part of the sacrum and then extends all the way across to attach to an area of the leg bone just before it becomes the hip joint.

This muscle provides an important function in the lower body because it stabilizes the hip joint and helps rotate the thigh muscle away from the body. The sciatic nerve, which combines the lower lumbar nerves and the first sacral nerve (L4, L5, and S1), either passes next to or actually goes through the piriformis muscle. When the piriformis muscle is inflamed, it will create pain in the buttock or cause pain, numbness, and tingling in the leg if the inflamed muscle irritates the sciatic nerve. Running and sitting for extended periods of time may trigger this pain. Most cases of sciatica and buttock pain, however, are due to an issue with the lumbar spine and *not* the piriformis muscle.

Strains and tears of the hamstring muscles can also cause buttock pain. The muscles that make up the hamstring all attach to the bottom of the pelvic bone. These muscles come together at a common area and fuse into one tendon where they attach to the pelvis (**Picture 98**).

These muscles are important in any movement that propels the body forward, so problems with these muscles typically occur often in runners and other athletes. Many of the symptoms mimic the buttock and sciatic

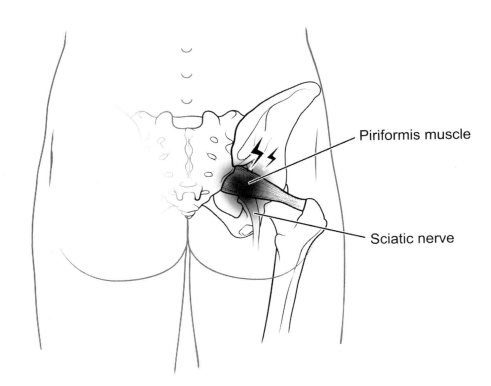

Piriformis muscle

Sciatic nerve

PICTURE 97

An inflamed piriformis muscle can create buttock pain.

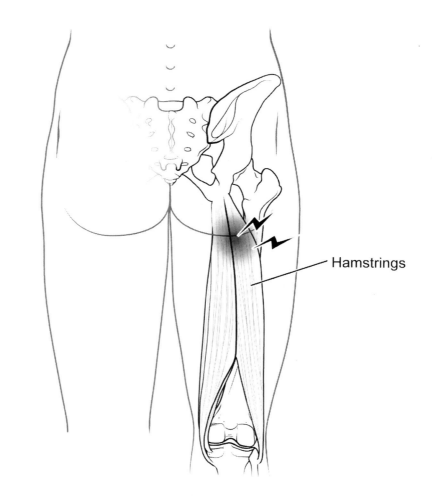

Hamstrings

PICTURE 98

Hamstring muscles where they attach to the pelvis can cause buttock pain when inflamed.

pain that you see when the problem is caused by the lumbar spine. In this case, buttock pain may radiate down the back of the leg, and the pain usually is worse when you sit or stretch the hamstring muscles. Remember, the sciatic nerve and the hamstring muscle run together down the back of the leg, so the pain may be similar. An MRI of the pelvis usually will show an area of inflammation or tear if the hamstring is involved. The therapy for hamstring pulls and tears is completely different from the treatment for pain coming from the lumbar nerve roots because of a problem in your back, and therefore you should get a diagnosis before therapy. In Chapter 17, I discuss the difference in therapy depending on whether the pain in the leg is due to the hamstring versus one of the lumbar nerve roots being inflamed. You do not want to stretch your hamstring muscle if the problem is coming from one of the lumbar nerve roots instead of the hamstring. This action may aggravate the lumbar nerve.

Arthritis and inflammation of the hip can be another cause of buttock pain. The hip joint is primarily in the front of the pelvis and creates more groin pain than pain in the buttock or the back of the pelvis **(Picture 99)**.

The hip may create discomfort very low in the buttock, almost at the same level as the lower pelvic bone to which the hamstring attaches **(Picture 100)**.

Picture 90 shows the different bones and muscles covered by the lumbar nerves. You will notice that a lot of the lumbar nerves (L3, L4, L5, and S1) can create pain in the *same* area as the hip joint, both in the low buttock area as well as the groin. Therefore, it is important to find out whether the lumbar spine or your hip is creating your groin or low buttock pain. A simple diagnostic hip block done under X-ray will quickly determine whether your hip joint is creating your buttock pain. Chapter 16 reviews the minimally invasive diagnostic procedures that can determine whether your pain is coming from your hip versus your lumbar spine.

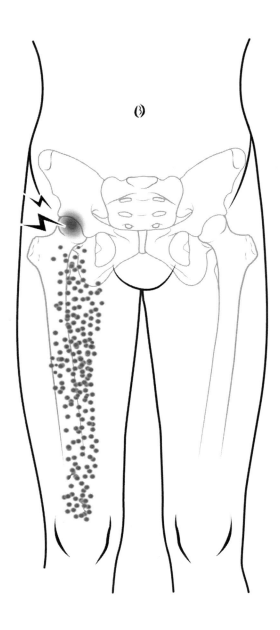

PICTURE 99

An inflamed hip joint usually creates groin pain and possible pain going down the front of the leg to the knee.

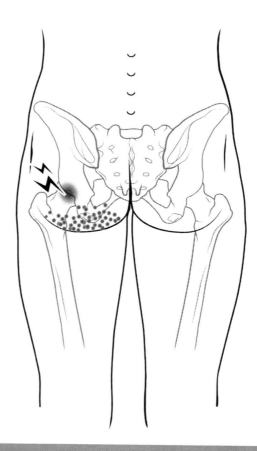

PICTURE 100

An inflamed hip joint can create pain in the low buttock area.

SUMMARY

1. The most common reason for buttock pain is an inflammation of the lumbar nerves.

2. The inflammation of the lumbar nerves can be due to a disc herniation, foraminal stenosis, or central spinal stenosis.

3. Inflammation of the hip joint can cause buttock pain.

4. An inflamed sacroiliac joint can create buttock pain, but it is not very common.

5. A strain or tear of the piriformis muscle or the hamstring muscle may cause buttock pain.

6. Always use a minimally invasive diagnostic procedure to diagnose your pain before treatment! This has to be done using X-ray guidance or possibly ultrasound.

7. Chapters 2 and 3 provide information about the lumbar spine.

8. Chapter 16 discusses the minimally invasive diagnostic procedures that I use to diagnose and treat buttock pain.

9. Chapter 17 provides information on therapy and exercises for the lumbar spine.

CHAPTER 13

My Tailbone Hurts When I Sit

Pain in the area of the coccyx, which is also called the tailbone, is called coccydynia. **Picture 101** shows the area of the body where patients with coccydynia feel pain.

The coccyx is the last bone in the human spine, and it is attached to the bone called the sacrum. Underneath the coccyx is a set of nerves called the Ganglion of Impar, which can become inflamed and create pain (**Picture 102**).

The usual symptom of an inflamed coccyx is pain in the tailbone area on sitting, but some patients notice that their tailbone is painful when they stand and walk. There is usually not a specific reason why the area around the coccyx bone starts to hurt, but an inflamed coccyx can be caused by some form of trauma or constant pressure on the tailbone. Coccydynia has been reported after childbirth, falling on the tailbone, or long periods of bicycle or horseback riding. All these activities can create an inflammation of the coccyx or the nerves right under the coccyx. Tumors of the coccyx

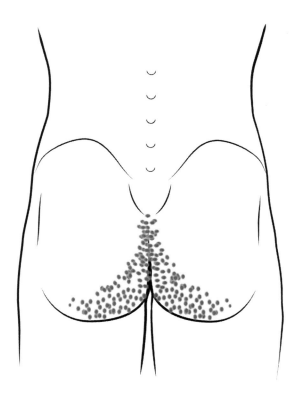

PICTURE 101

Area of pain created by inflammation of the coccyx.

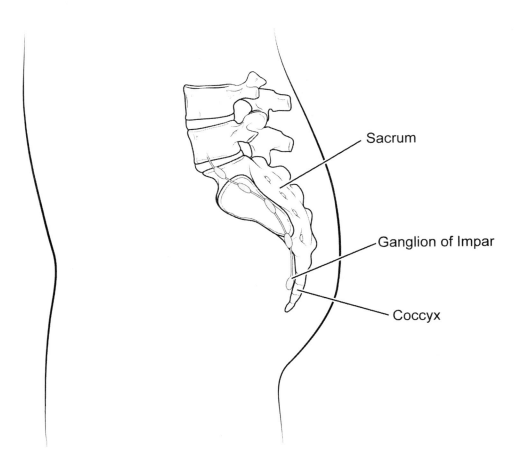

Coccyx and the
Ganglion of Impar.

and pelvis also can create pain in this area. I always order an X-ray and/or MRI of the pelvis before treating coccydynia.

If you have coccydynia you will notice that your tailbone will be tender to light touch and will hurt whenever you sit for any period of time. Many patients show up at my office carrying a cushion to sit on because of the pain. Coccydynia can be treated successfully with an injection of local anesthetic and steroids around the Ganglion of Impar. This procedure is discussed in Chapter 16.

Inflammation of the nerves of the lumbar and sacral part of the spine that go down into the area of the coccyx also can create pain in the coccyx area. A disc herniation or a condition called spinal stenosis, which involves a narrowing of the central canal, can irritate the nerves that go into the tailbone area. Pain in the tailbone area that is due to the inflammation of the lumbar and sacral nerves usually gets worse upon walking, but it can occur while sitting. This area of the coccyx usually is not tender to palpation because this is referred pain from the lumbar and sacral nerves and is not an actual problem with the tailbone. This can be an easy way to differentiate between pain coming from the lumbar spine and from the coccyx. Pain in the area of the tailbone will get better once the disc herniation or stenosis of the lumbar spine is treated.

SUMMARY

1. Pain in the tailbone area is called coccydynia and usually is most severe in the sitting position.

2. Trauma to the tailbone or constant pressure on the tailbone can create this type of pain, but usually there is no specific reason why coccydynia occurs.

3. Tumors of the coccyx and pelvis should be ruled out before treating the tailbone and the set of nerves, called the Ganglion of Impar, under the coccyx.

4. Coccydynia can be treated successfully by an injection of local anesthetic and steroids around the Ganglion of Impar.

5. The minimally invasive diagnostic procedure for coccydynia is discussed in Chapter 16.

My Groin Hurts

The groin is an area of the body that most people do not associate with the spine or musculoskeletal system. By the time I see the patient, the usual causes of groin pain such as hernias, male and female genitourinary issues, and other intra-abdominal conditions will have been ruled out.

The three most common causes of groin pain, as it relates to the musculoskeletal system, are hip bursitis or arthritis, tears or strains of one or more groin muscles, and lumbar nerve pain.

One of the most common causes of groin pain is hip bursitis or arthritis. The hip joint is located in the front of the pelvis and *not* in the area of the buttock, as you can see in **Picture 103**. Because the joint is located in the front part of the pelvis, if the pain is coming from the hip, one of the most common types of pain is groin pain. If your hip joint is creating the groin pain, the pain also may be in the front of the leg. The pain from the hip that goes down the leg never goes past the knee, and it is always in the *front* of the leg.

You also may have pain in the *very bottom* of the buttock, as the back of the hip joint is located in that area (**Picture 104**).

The hip joint is *not* located in the top or the middle of the buttock, just in the very bottom area where the buttock meets the leg. A lot of patients tell me that their hip is hurting while pointing to their buttock. Read Chapter 12 on buttock pain to get more information if your pain is primarily in the buttock.

Groin pain coming from the hip usually gets worse when standing or walking, and feels better when sitting down. To see whether the hip is creating the discomfort, sit down and cross the leg on the side where the groin hurts over the other leg (**Picture 105**).

If you notice that this position creates significant groin pain, then the pain very possibly is coming from the hip joint. An X-ray or an MRI usually will help confirm the diagnosis, but the MRI is not always diagnostic. For example, just because the MRI shows a degenerated hip does not mean your pain is coming from the hip joint. A lot of people just have age-related degeneration of their hip joint, which will show up on the MRI, but the hip is not creating the pain. I diagnose this problem by placing local anesthetic

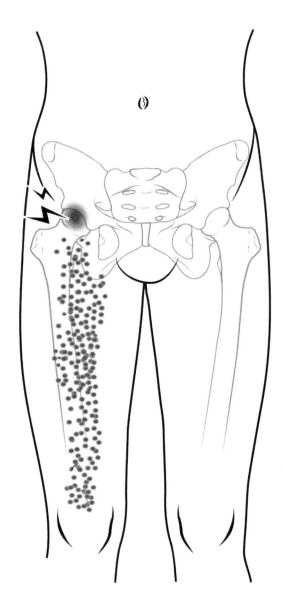

Pain in the groin due to inflammation in the hip joint.

inside the hip joint using an X-ray machine. This will give me an answer very quickly, as the local anesthetic takes only a short while to numb the inside of the joint. If the pain is gone after the local anesthetic is placed in the hip joint, you will know that the pain is coming from your hip joint. If you still have groin pain, then you know that your hip joint is not creating the groin pain.

Tears or strains of one or more groin muscles are another common cause of groin pain. Multiple muscles originate in the pelvis and attach to the inner side of the thighbone, otherwise called the femur. This type of groin injury usually occurs with some type of athletic activity, and it creates pain and swelling in the area of the inner thigh. The area also may be tender to palpation and appear to be bruised. Pain occurs when the patient tries to extend the leg outward away from the body and then bring it back toward the midline. The tear or strain usually shows up on an MRI.

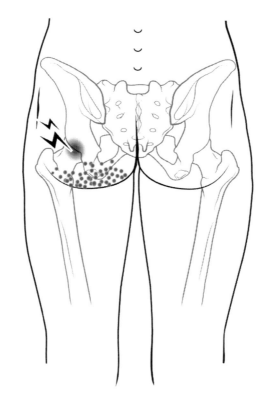

PICTURE 104

Pain in the lower area
of the buttock due to
inflammation in the
hip joint.

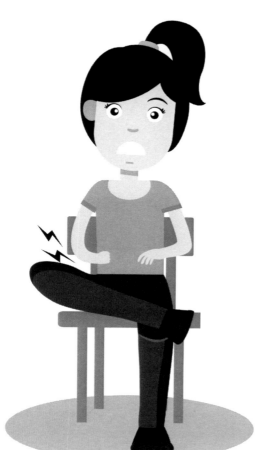

PICTURE 105

Crossing your leg to
see whether it creates
groin pain.

The third common cause of groin pain is lumbar nerve pain. *All* the nerves that originate in the lumbar spine can create groin pain. **Picture 106** shows the L1 and L2 nerves in the lumbar spine that cover the surface of the groin area. The T11 and T12 nerves also descend down to the groin. Therefore, you may notice groin pain if one of these nerves is inflamed because of a disc herniation or because the hole from which the nerve exits is narrowed.

Picture 107 shows where the lumbar nerves go to the *muscles* and *bones* of the groin area. As you can see, the L3, L4, L5, and S1 nerves cover the muscles and bones in the area of the groin, and therefore these nerves may create the groin pain.

If you combine Pictures 106 and 107, you now see that *all* of the lumbar nerves (L1, L2, L3, L4, L5, and S1) can create groin pain.

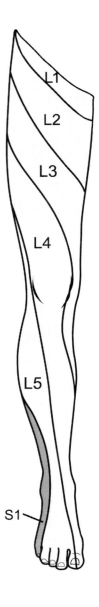

PICTURE 106

Lumbar nerves can create pain in the area of the groin when they are inflamed.

At times the answer to your groin pain may not be clear. For example, you may notice that you have groin and thigh pain, but you also may have some back pain. The question is whether the main source of pain is coming from the back or the hip. In those situations, minimally invasive diagnostic blocks of the structure in question easily provide an answer. If you have an X-ray–directed block of the hip joint with a local anesthetic and immediately afterward are able to walk and cross your leg without any pain, you then know that the source of the pain is your hip joint. If not, you know that

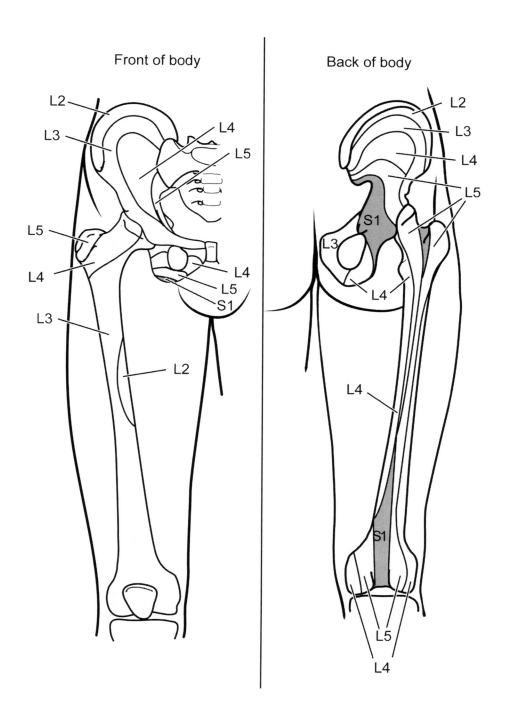

PICTURE 107

Lumbar nerves can create pain in the muscles and bones of the groin when they are inflamed.

your pain probably is coming from one of your lumbar nerves. Then your doctor can use a minimally invasive procedure to diagnose and treat the lumbar nerves.

SUMMARY

1. *All* the nerves of the lumbar spine can create groin pain.

2. You may or may not have discomfort in your back with the groin pain, even if the pain is coming from one of the nerves of the lumbar spine.

3. Consider the lower back as a cause of groin pain, especially if the hip joint and the groin muscles do not appear to be the source of the pain.

4. Chapters 2 and 3 provide more information on hip and lumbar nerve pain.

5. Chapter 16 discusses the minimally invasive procedures that are used to diagnose and treat groin pain.

PART III

Treatment and Care

CHAPTER 15

Which Medications Can I Try?

The use of medications for the treatment of spine pain can vary, whether prescribed for an intense, acute flare-up of pain over several weeks or for a longer-lasting, chronic condition of spine pain. The beauty of the human spine is that in most cases the acute, severe pain will diminish over the first few weeks. Your body will eliminate the inflammation around the structure in the spine that is creating your pain. At times, pain medications may be needed to control the pain while the body spontaneously heals itself over the first four to six weeks. Specific patient populations—for example, patients with cancer or severely degenerated spines—may need to be on some level of long-term medication management because of extenuating circumstances.

The main goal is to eliminate pain, either by using medications to give your body time to heal or by finding the specific inflamed structure in the spine or musculoskeletal system that is creating your pain. If your pain continues for longer than four to six weeks, the key to caring for spine and musculoskeletal pain is to find a diagnosis and then specifically to treat that structure so that the inflammation subsides. If this treatment is not successful, surgery should be considered.

AVOID LONG-TERM NARCOTICS

Quite often, the specific structure that is creating pain is *never* located, and therefore the pain never subsides. The next step for many physicians is to start patients on narcotics. Once patients are on narcotics and start developing a tolerance to medications, it is difficult either to wean them off the medication or to make a clear diagnosis. What may start out as an appropriate use of highly addicting pain medication and muscle relaxants for the treatment of an acute flare-up of intense back or neck pain can turn into years of continued use of these same medications for chronic back, neck, leg, or arm pain.

> **Remember: Do not allow yourself to start as a patient with acute spine pain and end by becoming a chronic pain patient!**

Spine pain is never constant, and in most cases, the severe pain will diminish over several weeks, as the body eliminates the inflammation around the structure in the spine. During this acute phase of the pain, a combination of anti-inflammatories, muscle relaxants, and even low-grade pain medications may be used to control the pain. If the pain does not subside, I will then use a minimally invasive diagnostic procedure to locate and eliminate the inflammation of the specific structure that is creating the pain. Chapter 16 will explain these procedures in detail. Always try to locate the source of your pain instead of masking it with narcotics!

MEDICATIONS FOR SPINE PAIN

Let me highlight the different categories of medications that I find useful for spine pain. Each medical practitioner may have a different way to medically manage spine pain, and there are many drugs that are used for pain, so do not look at this as a complete list or as the only way to treat spine pain. I would also recommend reading more about each one of these medications as there may be side effects and drug interactions that are specific for each person.

Nonsteroidal Anti-Inflammatory Drugs

Nonsteroidal anti-inflammatory drugs (NSAIDs) relieve inflammation and pain. All NSAIDs work in the same manner by blocking certain chemicals in the body that can create inflammation. Nonprescription versions of these medications usually contain either ibuprofen or naproxen. Some NSAIDs are available only with a prescription. There is not much difference in efficacy between nonprescription and prescription NSAIDs, except that the prescription types of medications may have a slow-release form or a higher strength that allows you to take them less often. The short-term use of any NSAID medication has been shown to be effective in patients with acute back pain. The long-term daily use of these medications for chronic back pain is not advocated because of possible side effects. I usually recommend this group of medications for acute back pain for short periods of time on an as-needed basis. That means you take these drugs only when you hurt, instead of taking them every day whether or not you hurt.

Steroidal Anti-Inflammatory Drugs

Steroidal anti-inflammatory drugs are used to relieve acute inflammation and therefore pain. They are considered more powerful than NSAIDs and usually are reserved for patients who do not obtain relief from NSAIDs. Oral steroids for spine pain should be used for very short periods of time. I usually place patients on them for five or six days and then discontinue use, whether or not the patient improves. Few side effects are associated with short-term use of oral steroids, but a number of complications have been associated with long-term use, including weight gain, osteoporosis, and stomach ulcers, to name a few. Diabetes may be a potential contraindication to the use of oral steroids because they can cause an increase in blood sugar. Steroids should not be used during an active infection, because the steroids can decrease your immunity and therefore keep you from healing.

Muscle Relaxants

Muscle relaxants are commonly used to treat muscle spasm during the initial phase of spine pain. This group of medications has been shown to be effective in the management of bouts of acute back pain, but not for chronic back pain. Some of the muscle relaxants have been shown to have a potential for drug dependence (addiction) and therefore should be monitored carefully and stopped after four to six weeks. Most muscle relaxants may have a sedating effect, so be careful when you first use them, as your body may need time to adjust.

Tramadol

Tramadol is a pain medication that has a mechanism of action that works similarly to a combination of three different medications: acetaminophen, an anti-depressant, and a narcotic. Even though it is a narcotic, it has a lower level of abuse and addiction potential than other narcotics. Tramadol is often used along with an anti-inflammatory medication to control the discomfort during the first four to six weeks. It can also be used for managing chronic pain on an as-needed basis.

Narcotics

The most common narcotics prescribed for pain are called opioids, which have some form of codeine mixed with acetaminophen. The two forms of codeine that are used for pain are Tylenol #3®, which has 30 mg of codeine, and Tylenol #4®, which has 60 mg of codeine. Two opioids that use synthetic codeine are hydrocodone and oxycodone. Hydrocodone, which is the generic name for Vicodin® and Norco®, usually is mixed with either acetaminophen or ibuprofen in various strengths and is used for acute back pain. You need to understand how these medications compare to each other. For example, 30 mg of codeine (Tylenol #3) is going to provide about the same pain relief as 5 mg hydrocodone, and 60 mg of codeine (Tylenol #4) is about the same strength as 10 mg of hydrocodone. One 10 mg tablet of hydrocodone (Vicodin, Norco) provides the same amount of narcotic as more than 5 mg of morphine. So if you take three tablets of the 10 mg of hydrocodone a day, you essentially are taking 15 mg of morphine a day. Many people, including medical personnel, fail to appreciate the strength of these narcotics, which is why some of the stronger pain medications are frequently prescribed without trying the less potent medications first. This is also why many practitioners continue prescribing these narcotics long-term without understanding their effect on the human body.

Two things occur when you take narcotics for a long period of time. First, the body develops a significant tolerance for narcotics, which means that you have to keep taking higher doses of the narcotic to get the same effect, and second, your body will develop a hypersensitivity to pain, which means that your perception of your pain will change: your pain will feel like it is a lot worse than it really is. Both of these effects should be a signal to your medical practitioner to consider weaning you off narcotic medications. Unfortunately, the opposite usually occurs, and medical practitioners frequently increase the dose of the narcotics. *Do not allow yourself to go down this path!* You are better off locating the problem in your spine that is creating your pain instead of taking long-term narcotics.

Neuropathic Medications

Neuropathic medications are well known for their abilities to decrease the pain that comes from nerves. The nerves in your spine may be inflamed or injured because of the irritation of the disc, the narrowing of the spinal canal, or scar tissue. Symptoms associated with nerve pain include numbness, tingling, burning, and shooting pain. The two drugs that are commonly used are gabapentin (Neurontin®) or pregabalin (Lyrica®). These drugs have been shown to be more beneficial for nerve pain than narcotics. Neuropathic drugs slow the impulses traveling down the nerve instead of just masking the pain. This group of drugs can be used in combination with other medications to provide good relief without having to use potent narcotics. For example, combining tramadol and gabapentin will provide relief from lower back muscle or bone pain as well as the nerve pain.

WHICH MEDICATIONS TO USE DEPENDING ON THE DURATION OF YOUR PAIN

Following is a time frame for medications that I recommend for spine pain depending on the onset of your discomfort. I mention a few other things you can do along with taking the medications to help you control the pain. Again, most spine pain will resolve on its own in four to six weeks. You are merely buying time to give your body a chance to heal.

From Onset to Four Weeks

Start with an over-the-counter anti-inflammatory NSAID such as ibuprofen or naproxen. You can also use ice or heat on the affected area depending on which works better for you. Be careful with heat as you can burn your skin. If the pain is so severe that the over-the-counter medication does not get the job done, it is time to see a medical practitioner. I usually start with a longer-acting NSAID or a trial of oral steroids at this time. I may add tramadol to help with the pain until the NSAIDs or steroids can eradicate the inflammation. Depending on the severity of the pain, I may add acetaminophen with codeine and/or one of the neuropathic medications. Physical therapy, chiropractic treatment, acupuncture, and continued exercise are excellent ways to deal with the discomfort during this period. Read Chapter 17 on therapy and exercises that may help with your pain as well as teach you how to stay active and exercise without aggravating your discomfort. Staying active is good, but you should not do things that create pain. For example, if bending forward hurts, don't do yoga exercises that make you bend forward. If arching your back hurts, don't do physical therapy exercises that involve doing that type of movement. If walking hurts, do not walk much, as you are aggravating the problem that is creating your pain. When you do something that creates pain, your body is telling you that you are actually aggravating something, not helping it heal.

Four to Six Weeks

If you are still hurting after four to six weeks, but are getting better, I would recommend that you start to wean off the more potent narcotics if you are taking one at this time. I will usually continue the tramadol and an NSAID on an as-needed basis and then stop them as the pain continues to subside. If you are not getting better at this point and are still having to use narcotic pain medications on a regular basis, or are having issues with your daily activities, it may be time to locate the source of your pain. Chapter 16 will show you how to find the structure in the spine that is creating the pain and eradicate the inflammation at the same time.

Six Weeks or Longer

After six weeks or more, if you are doing well or just have a few sporadic episodes of pain, go to Chapter 17 and skip the rest of this book. If you are not getting better, read Chapter 16 because it will show you how to diagnose and treat the issue that is creating your pain. Some patients will choose to stay on medications and not go down the path of diagnostic or therapeutic procedures. For that group, the use of tramadol on an as-needed basis and the neuropathic medications are best for pain management depending on the type of pain you are suffering from. The use of other narcotics should be sporadic at best, and *only* during severe flare-ups of pain. You should *not* continue using narcotics every day without seeking an answer. Extended use of narcotics will just increase your tolerance of the drugs, leading you to keep raising your intake, and also increase your sensitivity to pain, so your feeling of pain increases at the same time! This is exactly how patients go from having some form of acute pain to becoming a chronic pain patient. You are better off locating and treating the structure that is creating your problem.

> **Remember: Do not allow temporary pain to become chronic pain!**

SUMMARY

1. Spine pain is usually temporary, as most of the acute discomfort subsides over a period of four to six weeks. During this time, the use of pain medications, muscle relaxants, and anti-inflammatories is warranted.

2. Narcotic pain medications should be used only sporadically for acute severe pain and should be stopped at four to six weeks.

3. The specific inflamed structure in the spine should be located and treated if the pain continues for longer than four to six weeks.

4. Chapter 16 discusses the minimally invasive procedures that are used to locate and treat the inflamed structure.

5. Chapter 17 provides information about therapy to help you manage your pain and shows you exercises to do once your pain has resolved.

Minimally Invasive Procedures That Give You Answers

THE BASIS FOR MINIMALLY INVASIVE PROCEDURES

Twenty percent of patients who started to have spine pain will continue to have discomfort even though they may have tried medication management, physical therapy, home exercises, chiropractor care, acupuncture, or maybe just living with the pain while they waited for it to subside. If your pain is still bothering you, the usual next step is a minimally invasive procedure.

The minimally invasive procedures that I perform are always done using a continuous X-ray machine. All pictures that are taken by the X-ray machine are saved and become part of the report. A mixture of local anesthetic and steroids is placed on the spinal structure through a needle while the patient is lightly sedated. The local anesthetic numbs the structure, and immediately after the procedure I evaluate the patient to see if the pain has been eliminated. If I have located the right structure, the pain will be gone. This is the diagnostic part of the injection. The steroid that is mixed with the local anesthetic will begin to work within a couple of days, but it may take up to two or three weeks after the injection is given for the steroid to peak. This is the long-term therapeutic part of the injection.

Minimally invasive procedures are designed to do three things:

1. Help determine the cause of your pain.

2. Eliminate the inflammation.

3. Possibly provide long-term relief.

Help Determine the Cause of the Pain

In a lot of situations, the patient's symptoms and the physical exam do not give a clear-cut diagnosis, or the symptoms do not match the MRI findings. As we age, our spine and joints will continue to degenerate, and those changes will show up on the MRI; however, in the majority of cases, we will not experience pain due to the degeneration.

> **Remember: An MRI does not show pain, just wear and tear. As people age, they develop degenerated joints and herniated discs that create no pain. Do not use just an MRI to make a diagnosis!**

Pain from the disc herniation or joint is usually secondary to an inflammatory response. And the pain has nothing to do with the size of the disc or how arthritic the joint is. For example, let's say you have a large disc herniation in your lumbar spine at one level that is not inflamed, and a smaller disc herniation at another that is inflamed. The MRI is not going to tell you which one is creating your pain. You need a minimally invasive diagnostic procedure to tell you which one is creating your pain.

Here is another common problem that I see all the time. A patient will come to me with pain in the shoulder area and an MRI that shows some wear and tear inside the shoulder joint. An MRI of the neck shows a herniated disc at C4-C5 that is pressing on the C5 nerve, which is the nerve that covers the area of the shoulder. This patient will need a diagnostic procedure to determine whether it is the shoulder joint or the neck that is creating pain over the area of the shoulder. I use a minimally invasive diagnostic procedure to pinpoint the specific problem that is creating the pain.

Let us go over the two examples that I just gave in order to see how the minimally invasive procedure gives you diagnostic information. If you are the patient with the two disc herniations, one large and the other one small, you face a dilemma of trying to determine which one is creating the pain. Using a quick-acting local anesthetic, I would numb the nerve that runs by the disc that comes closest to matching your pain diagram and your symptoms—*not* the largest disc herniation, but the one that is most likely creating your pain. If your pain is gone right after the procedure, I would then know that the smaller disc is creating your pain. If the pain persisted, I would then numb the nerve that runs by the other disc to see whether the pain was eliminated. This type of diagnostic approach ensures that if you need surgery, you can be sure that the right disc is operated on.

The next example is the patient who has pain in the shoulder, and the patient and the physician are trying to figure out whether it is inflammation inside the shoulder joint or one of the nerves in the cervical spine that is creating the shoulder pain. The two types of shoulder pain can be very similar whether the pain is coming from the shoulder or the neck. You can get an exact diagnosis through minimally invasive diagnostic procedures. I would numb the inside of the shoulder joint, and if the shoulder pain is gone immediately after the procedure, then you know that the pain is coming from the shoulder. If the pain persists, then I would numb the nerve in the neck and see whether the pain went away. This is a simple way to arrive at a diagnosis. This type of information is essential since it can be used to help make decisions on the type of therapy, possible surgery, and daily life changes that need to be made. Do you do physical therapy for the neck or the shoulder? Do you need to be careful about how you use your shoulder? Or how you use your neck? Should anybody operate on your shoulder when your pain is coming from the neck?

Eliminate the Inflammation

Minimally invasive procedures are used not only to locate the structure that is creating the pain, but also to eliminate the inflammation and subsequently the discomfort. The minimally invasive diagnostic procedures are performed with a combination of a quick-acting local anesthetic and a steroidal anti-inflammatory agent. The local anesthetic works immediately and gives a diagnostic answer, as was just discussed. The steroidal anti-inflammatory agent gives the long-term relief. It can take two to three weeks for the steroidal anti-inflammatory agent that is mixed with the local anesthetic to take effect. *There is no long-term masking effect from the procedure.* I highlight this point because I get this question all the time. The only masking effect is from the diagnostic local anesthetic and that effect is gone in several hours. If you re-aggravate the structure, your pain will return.

Provide Long-Term Relief

Two questions always come up when discussing long-term relief: How long? And how come? Patients want to know how long the relief will last and how can long-term relief be achieved if you still have herniated, degenerated discs and arthritic facet joints.

In answer to the first question, results can vary from many years to a few weeks. I have had patients that I have treated once and came back to see me years later for a different problem, and I have seen patients who got only a few weeks of relief and subsequently required surgery. All patients have their own opinion of what long-term relief means to them, but I personally have had diagnostic minimally invasive injections in both the lumbar and cervical areas, and I got anywhere from months to many years of relief. At times, I have had to have two injections within a month or two before the inflammation and pain went away. I have noticed that my relief from the procedures has gotten longer since I made significant changes in my activities to keep the structures in my spine from becoming re-inflamed too quickly. I quit playing basketball and tennis and instead started swimming and bike riding. Chapter 17 explains how to avoid the return of pain by working on your body mechanics and exercises so that you do not re-inflame the structure in your spine that was creating your pain.

How can long-term relief be achieved if you still have disc herniations, arthritic joints, and all sorts of changes in your spine? The answer is the beauty of the human body!

Most people will hurt only if the herniated disc, nerve, or facet is *inflamed*.

> **Remember: A lot of herniated discs and arthritic changes in your spine will never create pain. The simple reason is that pain usually occurs only in the presence of inflammation, not degeneration. So if the spinal diagnostic procedure eliminates the inflammation, you can obtain long-term relief even though you still have herniated discs and arthritic changes in your spine.**

Obtaining long-term relief is possible *as long as* you do not re-aggravate the area of degeneration and create more inflammation. This is not as easy as it sounds, as basic things that you do in life, such as driving to work, mowing the yard, or the weekend game of golf, may be enough to create a re-aggravation of the degenerated area. Some patients have jobs or activities that prevent them from changing their lifestyles. I stress to patients that their pain will return not when the steroids wear off, which is only in a couple of weeks, but when they re-aggravate their spine! You can prolong the relief of the procedure by learning better body mechanics, exercising, and changing a few things in the way you work or play. If you read Chapter 17 and learn how to change your lifestyle and body mechanics, you may be able to keep your spine from getting re-aggravated and re-inflamed. At times, however, the compression of the nerves in the spine is severe, or the inflammation will not go away, and the only way to fix the problem is to have surgery.

THE MINIMALLY INVASIVE DIAGNOSTIC PROCEDURES

Now that you know the basis for the minimally invasive procedures, you need to know a few more things before you have a procedure done:

1. A well-trained physician should do the procedure. This person should not just be an anesthesiologist or physical medicine physician, but someone who has received at least six months to a year of additional fellowship training after residency. This does not mean weekend training courses.

2. These procedures *must* be done with the use of an X-ray machine. The structures that we are trying to locate to see if they are creating your pain can be accurately located *only* with the benefit of an X-ray machine.

3. The pictures of the X-rays that are taken during the procedure *must* be saved and filed with your chart. Insurance companies should ask physicians who do these procedures to send a copy of the X-rays to the

company, as this is the only way that the exact procedure that was done can be documented. Many patients that I see tell me that they have already had a "spine procedure" done that produced only minimal relief, but there were *no* X-ray pictures to show the exact location of the spine that was treated. A lot of these same patients get better after I treat them. What does that tell you? Did the physician really do the procedure that was supposed to be done? Or was there a different area that needed to be treated instead? Make sure you get the X-ray copy of your procedure once it is done!

4.   The amount of relief immediately after the procedure *must* be documented. This is essential because it gives you the diagnostic information that will be needed if you do not get long-term relief. The local anesthetic that is used for these procedures will wear off in several hours, so I make sure that patients stay active during that time so they can assess their level of pain.

5.   The patient should *not* be on large doses of oral narcotics or be given narcotics during the sedation process of the procedure, if the procedure is diagnostic. Narcotics will eliminate the diagnostic part of the procedure, which is essential.

6.   The steroid that is injected at the same time the local anesthetic is placed on the nerve, disc, or facet joint can take *two to three weeks* to reach its full effect in eliminating the inflammation. Do not have a repeat procedure done for at least three weeks because you may not notice relief until the end of the second or third week.

Only a few procedures are used to diagnose and treat most spine pain. If you have read the earlier chapters in this book, you would now realize that only three structures in the spine create most of the pain when they are inflamed: the disc, the facet, and the nerve.

Picture 108 shows these three structures of the spine along with the procedures that are used to treat them when they are inflamed. The inflamed structures are seen on the left and the procedures on the right.

Depending on which structure is inflamed, I usually perform one of the following three procedures:

1.   An intradiscal steroid injection if the inside of the disc is inflamed.

2.   A nerve root block if a herniated disc is inflaming the nerve.

3.   A facet block if the facet joint is irritated.

Let's discuss each one of these procedures so that you may have a better idea of what they are and what they treat. The most important thing to realize is that not all injections are the same, so you cannot just treat every back

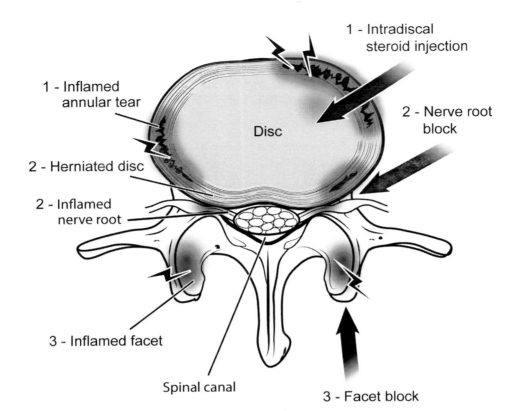

1 - Intradiscal steroid injection

1 - Inflamed annular tear

Disc

2 - Nerve root block

2 - Herniated disc

2 - Inflamed nerve root

3 - Inflamed facet

Spinal canal

3 - Facet block

PICTURE 108

Procedures used in treating inflamed structures in the spine.

or neck pain with the *same* injection and expect to have good relief. You cannot expect to use a procedure that treats the facets if your back pain is coming from the disc. I will talk about this later in the chapter.

Nerve Root Block

The most common procedure that I perform is the nerve root block, which is a placement of local anesthetic and steroids directly around the nerve that is inflamed. These nerves are found in every part of the spine, starting from the cervical area, through the thoracic spine, down to the lumbar and sacral spine. The nerve roots are the nerves that run by the disc and out the holes in the spine. This procedure primarily is used to eliminate the inflammation of the nerve because of a disc herniation or because of the narrowing of the hole from which the nerve exits the spine (foraminal stenosis). **Picture 109** shows the local anesthetic and steroid medication being placed directly on the nerve. The local anesthetic works very quickly and gives diagnostic information. If your pain is gone right after I do this procedure, then I know I have located the problem creating your pain. The steroids can take several weeks to eliminate the inflammation and the pain. A second injection may be given about three weeks after the first procedure if the patient does not obtain complete relief.

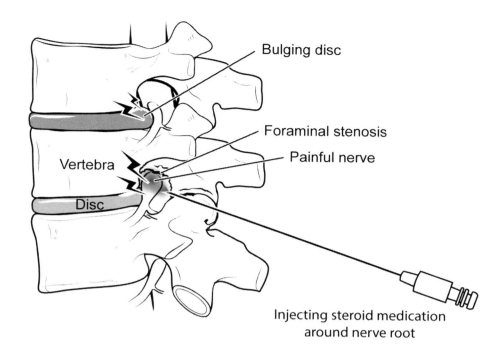

Nerve root injection of local anesthetic and steroids.

Facet Joint Block and Facet Joint Radiofrequency Thermocoagulation (RFTC)

The facet block is an injection of local anesthetic and steroids that is placed into the capsule of the inflamed facet joint, the same way you treat an inflamed knee or shoulder joint **(Picture 110)**. This procedure is used to diagnose and treat inflamed facet joints. The facets, like the nerves, can be found at every level of the spine, from the cervical spine all the way down to the lumbar spine.

This procedure should only be done for back or neck pain without any leg or arm pain. If you have leg or arm pain, a nerve root block should be done because the facets do not create arm or leg pain. Most back or neck pain is created by the disc or nerve, not the facet. Therefore, even though you may have only back or neck pain, with no arm or leg pain, if you have degenerated or herniated discs in your spine, always consider those as the first possible source of your pain. Even when this procedure is done for the right reason, many physicians place the steroids not *into* the joint, but instead around the outside of the joint because it is easier to do. When you do not get long-term relief, the physician starts talking about burning the nerves around the joint. Demand a copy of your X-ray pictures, because this will force the physician to try to do the procedure the right way.

Radiofrequency thermocoagulation, also abbreviated as RFTC, is a common pain management procedure that involves "burning" the nerves that go to the facets. This procedure is also at times referred to as an "ablation of the nerves of the facet joints." The idea behind this procedure is to mask the pain

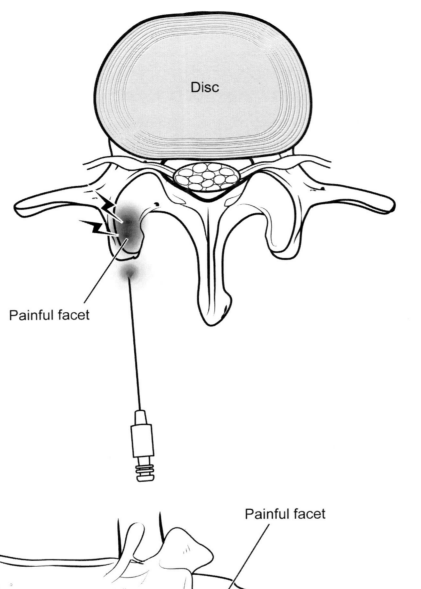

Disc

Painful facet

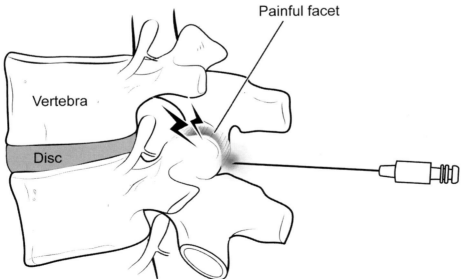

Painful facet

Vertebra

Disc

PICTURE 110

Facet joint injection of local anesthetic and steroids.

by destroying the nerves that go to the facet joints. The procedure is used when patients do not get long-term relief from facet blocks, meaning at least six months. Some facilities that do a lot of marketing on the Internet and television call RFTC a laser procedure, even though no laser is used.

I rarely have to do this procedure, for several reasons. The first is that most patients do not have facet pain, as most spine pain comes from the disc and the nerve. I frequently see patients who have pain going down their arms and legs, and they tell me that they have had an RFTC procedure with minimal relief. Facet pain cannot create pain going down the arms and legs! Only the nerves that come out of your spinal canal create that type of pain, and you *cannot* burn those nerves.

The second reason that I do not do many RFTC procedures is that most patients who truly have facet pain obtain good relief with facet blocks, if the steroid is actually placed *inside* the joint. You will not achieve long-term relief from a facet joint injection unless the steroid is placed correctly. If the steroids are placed not *inside* the facet joint but just around the *outside* of the facet, you will not get long-term benefits. And then you have to start burning nerves. And the last reason I do not like doing this procedure is that I do not like masking the pain from the facet joints by destroying the nerve that innervates the facet, especially in young, active patients. RFTC may be suitable for patients who do not get at least six months of pain relief from a facet block. The relief from RFTC can last anywhere from six months to several years, but the nerves from the facets can grow back.

Intradiscal Injection

Injection of the inside of the disc with local anesthetic and steroids is called an intradiscal injection (**Picture 111**). This procedure is used for inflammation that is coming from the *inside* of the disc. Placing steroids on the outside of the disc, either with a nerve root injection or an epidural steroid injection, will not get the job done if the inflammation is *inside* the disc. I have seen numerous patients who have had countless injections—epidurals, facet injections, sacroiliac joint injections, and trigger point injections—with no relief, because the patient had inflammation *inside* the disc, and the steroid was never placed *inside* the disc. A common symptom that reveals that your pain is possibly coming from inside the disc is your inability to sit for any length of time without having significant back pain. Read Chapter 4 to understand the pain that comes from inside the disc.

The rest of the procedures in this section are primarily therapeutic injections. There is minimal diagnostic information that can be obtained from them. A few of these procedures have a place in my practice, but only in certain specific situations.

Painful disc tears

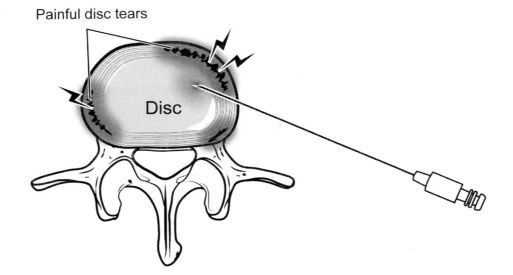

PICTURE 111

Intradiscal injection of steroid and local anesthetic.

Epidural Injection

The epidural steroid injection is an injection of steroids into the epidural space. It was at one time the most common procedure used for spine pain, as it could be done without the use of an X-ray machine. This procedure now should be used primarily to treat the pain from central spinal stenosis, because most nerve pain is better treated with nerve root blocks. The epidural steroid injection, which is placed into the area of the central stenosis, should always be done using X-ray guidance (**Picture 112**).

An epidural steroid injection is *not* the best choice for a disc herniation that is inflaming a specific nerve—for two reasons. First, as **Picture 113** shows, once the steroids are in the epidural space, the steroid and local anesthetic have to flow from the epidural space to the point at which the nerve runs by the disc herniation.

If the epidural space is obstructed by the disc, or if the hole from which the nerve exits is narrowed, the steroid may not get to the area of the nerve that is inflamed. The second reason that the epidural is not the best procedure for specific nerve pain is that the steroids can spread to many different nerves in the epidural space at the same time. Even if you do get relief for a short period of time, your pain may return, and you still do not know which nerve is creating your pain. The epidural is not a specific minimally invasive procedure. It is a pain management procedure with limited benefits. If your nerve pain is due to anything other than central stenosis, you should have a

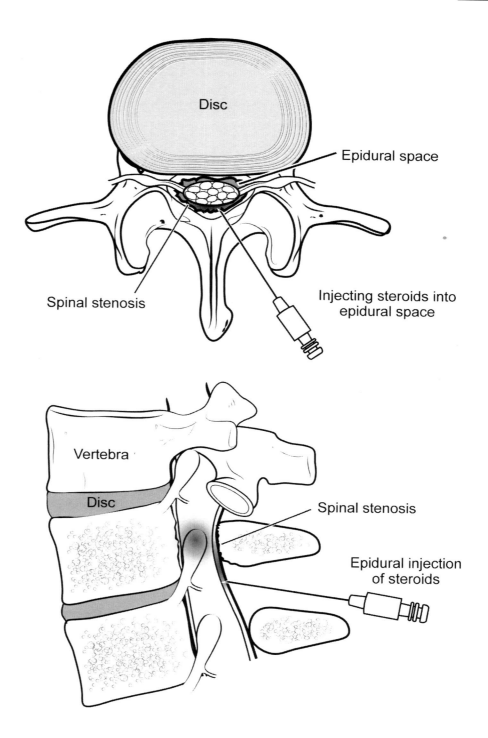

PICTURE 112

Epidural injection of steroids for spinal stenosis.

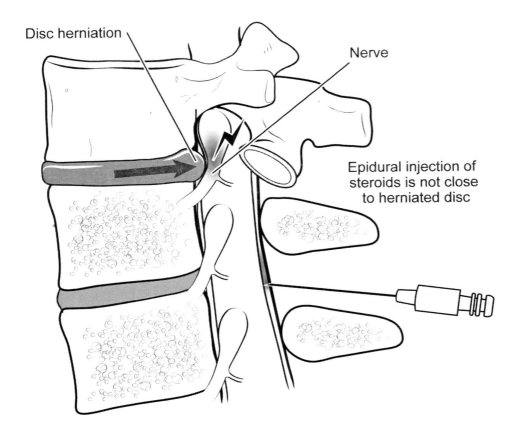

Disc herniation

Nerve

Epidural injection of steroids is not close to herniated disc

PICTURE 113

Epidural steroid injection is not the procedure of choice for disc herniations inflaming a specific nerve.

nerve root block instead of an epidural steroid injection. The epidural space usually is eliminated in patients who have had surgery, because surgeons have to make the incision through the epidural space, so, in those patients, a nerve root block will be far more effective than an epidural even for spinal stenosis. Two other important things you need to know about epidurals. The first is that a lot of medical practitioners will do an epidural steroid injection but call it a nerve root block. Always demand your X-ray pictures to make sure you are getting the correct procedure! The second is that physicians will do these procedures as a series of three injections, each one week apart. There is absolutely no reason to do this because it takes several weeks to get the full effect of the first injection. I would consider doing a second injection on a patient after three weeks only if the patient is still having pain.

Sacroiliac Joint Block

A sacroiliac joint block is used to treat the pain that comes from the inflammation of the sacroiliac joint, which is the joint between your sacrum and your pelvis (**Picture 114**). This procedure frequently is done when patients have buttock pain. Because most buttock pain actually originates from the lumbar nerves, I rarely do a sacroiliac joint block. Everything else that

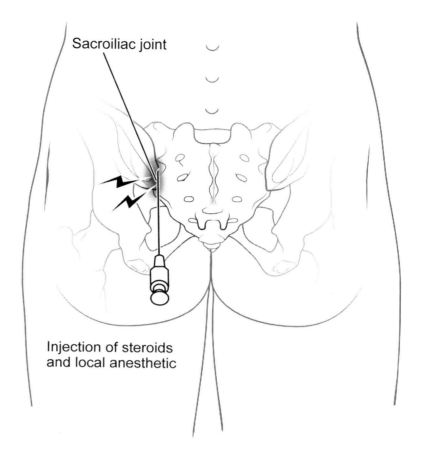

Sacroiliac joint

Injection of steroids
and local anesthetic

PICTURE 114

Sacroiliac joint
injection of steroids
and local anesthetic.

possibly could create buttock pain should be looked at before having this block. Make sure that this block is done using an X-ray machine, because it is impossible to do this procedure with a blind injection into the buttock. Always ask for the pictures of your procedure to confirm that whoever did the block actually got the medications into the joint. Read Chapter 12 for more information about pain in the buttock before having this procedure.

Ganglion of Impar Block and Coccyx Block

Ganglion of Impar and coccyx blocks are done for pain in the tailbone area. If the set of nerves under the tailbone is inflamed, it will create tailbone pain **(Picture 115)**. Placing a local anesthetic and steroids under the tailbone where the Ganglion of Impar is located may stop the inflammation in that area. Read Chapter 13 for information on pain in the tailbone area.

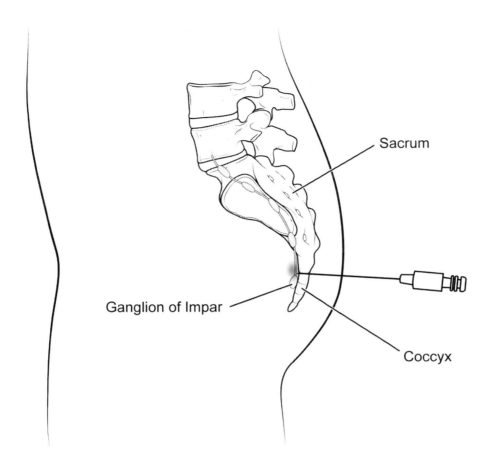

Sacrum

Ganglion of Impar

Coccyx

PICTURE 115

Ganglion of Impar
block.

HOW TO USE MINIMALLY INVASIVE PROCEDURES TO HELP DIAGNOSE YOUR PAIN

The easiest way to understand how these procedures are used to help diagnose and treat your pain is for me to review the different areas of pain that I have covered in the earlier chapters of this book, point out which structures are most likely to cause the pain, and then identify the best procedure to treat that problem. I do this to ensure that you receive the correct procedure for the right reason. By using a local anesthetic and a steroid in the injection, we accomplish two objectives: *locate the problem* and *eliminate the inflammation.*

My Back and/or Leg Hurts When I Sit, but Feels Better When I Walk (Chapter 4)

The two structures usually associated with this type of pain are the nerve and the disc, in that order. Using patient history, an exam, and an MRI usually narrows this down. I usually start with the lumbar nerve root block if the patient is having any pain in the hips and legs. I start by placing steroids inside the disc if the pain is only in the back and gets worse with sitting and better when you walk. Chapter 4 provides more information regarding pain that is coming from your nerve root or disc. Read Chapter 5 for more information about facet and spinal stenosis pain.

Lumbar nerve root block. The procedure is done to isolate the nerve that is creating the back pain and to provide relief by eliminating the inflammation. The most common lumbar nerve roots that create pain in the back and the leg are the L3, L4, L5, and S1 nerve roots.

Lumbar intradiscal steroid injection. This is the procedure of choice if the pain appears to be coming from inside the disc. The most common symptom of disc pain is significant back pain with sitting that feels better when you walk around. By placing dye in the disc, I can see the tears in the disc as well as obtain diagnostic information. This procedure is also a therapeutic way to treat the pain coming from *inside* the disc, because the steroid will reduce the inflammation. If the pain is coming from inside the disc, you never will eliminate the pain by placing medication just on the *outside* of the disc, which is what is done with the epidural and the nerve root block. This is a good example of how, with one procedure, you can locate the structure creating the problem and treat it at the same time. Any lumbar disc can create back pain, but the most common are the two bottom discs: L4-L5 and L5-S1.

My Back Keeps Me from Sleeping at Night and/or It Hurts to Stand in One Place (Chapter 5)

The two areas of the spine that usually create pain at night or when you stand in one place are the inflamed facets and narrowing of the spine (called spinal stenosis). Read Chapter 5 for more information about facet and spinal stenosis pain.

Lumbar facet block. Inflammation of the facet joint is a common problem that creates back pain while you are sleeping or standing upright as these positions cause inflamed facets to press on each other and create pain. This procedure is most effective in relieving facet joint pain if that is the source of your discomfort. It is done using an X-ray machine while placing a local anesthetic and steroids inside the facet joint. If the lumbar facets are the root of your problem, you will feel immediate relief as well as long-term relief within two to three weeks.

Lumbar epidural steroid injection. Spinal stenosis, the narrowing of the canal of the spine, also can create pain at night, as well as a stiff and sore back in the morning. If you have spinal stenosis, this happens because your spinal canal narrows when you lie flat in the bed. This narrowing of your canal can irritate the nerves inside the canal, which in turn can create back pain, hip and leg pain, and cramps in your legs. If you have spinal stenosis, you will tend to sleep on your side in a fetal position as this position will provide you relief by keeping your spinal canal open. The epidural attempts to remove the inflammation in the area of the spinal canal that is narrowed. The narrowing can occur at any level, so a combination of the clinical findings and the MRI will determine which areas need to be treated with the epidural. I usually do an epidural above and below the area of stenosis to try to get the steroids through the area that is narrowed. This procedure needs to be done with an X-ray machine to ensure coverage of the epidural space that is narrowed.

Lumbar nerve root block. If you have had surgery and the epidural space is no longer intact, the lumbar nerve root block is the best procedure to try to get the steroids into the area of narrowing. Practitioners are wasting their time if they cannot get the steroids to the area that is narrowed by doing an epidural in an area of previous surgery.

My Back and/or Legs Hurt When I Stand or Walk, but Feel Better When I Sit (Chapter 6)

The most common diagnosis for this complaint is lumbar spinal stenosis. Spinal stenosis is a narrowing of the spinal canal usually due to herniated discs or enlarged facet joints. Read Chapter 6 for more information about spinal stenosis.

Lumbar epidural. This is one procedure that is not diagnostic but may be therapeutic. An epidural steroid injection is probably the best procedure for central spinal stenosis. It allows the most anti-inflammatory steroid to move into the narrowed central part of the canal and can cover several levels in the spine. The epidural attempts to remove the inflammation in the area of the spinal canal that is narrowed. The narrowing can occur at any level, so the combination of the clinical findings and the MRI will help determine which areas need to be treated with the epidural. I usually do an epidural above and below the area of stenosis to try to get the steroids through the area that is narrowed. This procedure needs to be done with an X-ray machine to ensure coverage of the epidural space that is narrowed.

Lumbar facet block. I mention this procedure only because many patients have facet pain at the same time that they have pain from their spinal stenosis. The large arthritic facets actually cause the spinal stenosis. I usually treat the facets at the same time that I do the lumbar epidural steroid injection.

Lumbar nerve root block. If you have had surgery and the epidural space is no longer intact, the best procedure to try to get the steroids into the area of narrowing is the lumbar nerve root block. Not an epidural.

My Hip Hurts (Chapter 7)

This is a common complaint that is easily diagnosed. The pain usually comes from the hip or the nerves in the lower back. If you have any question about the source of your pain, I would suggest having these blocks done before surgery. The real beauty of minimally invasive diagnostic procedures is that in a patient with hip pain, you can arrive at a diagnosis very quickly, and in a lot of circumstances, the procedure may provide long-term relief if the pain is coming from one of the lumbar nerves. Even more important, once you have a diagnosis, you can plan treatment and therapy. Read Chapter 7 for more information about hip pain and for details about how the lumbar spine creates pain in the area of the hip.

Hip block. In a hip block, the local anesthetic and the anti-inflammatory medication are placed in the hip joint. This is done either by using an X-ray machine or an ultrasound machine to ensure that the medication really gets into the hip joint. The local anesthetic that is placed in the hip joint works in minutes. You should walk around right after the block and see whether the pain in your hip is gone. If the pain is coming from the hip joint, you should notice complete relief. If you still have discomfort, then you will know that the hip pain is probably coming from a nerve in the back. At that point, I move on to a lumbar nerve block, which is performed the same day.

Lumbar nerve root block. If the hip joint block does not eliminate the pain, and the block of the lumbar nerve gives you immediate relief, then you know that your hip pain actually is coming from your back.

My Shoulder Hurts—I Have Pain Around My Shoulder Blade (Chapter 8)

Pain in the *back* of the shoulder usually is due to one of the facets, discs, or nerves in the cervical spine and rarely is coming from the shoulder joint. The nerve or facet in the thoracic spine also can create pain into the back of the shoulder. If your pain also goes down the arm, then it is most likely the cervical nerve. Do not have someone do a cervical facet block on you if you have arm pain, because the facet never creates arm pain. Read Chapter 8 for more information regarding pain in the back of the shoulder.

Cervical nerve root block. This procedure is the exact same procedure as a lumbar nerve root block, but is done in the cervical spine instead. The nerve is treated with a local anesthetic and a steroid anti-inflammatory medication, and then assessed immediately afterward for relief. If pain in the back of the shoulder is gone, you have an answer to what has been creating your pain. The effect of the steroids may take a couple of weeks to completely kick in. The most common cervical nerve roots that create pain in the area of the back of the shoulder are the C5, C6, and C7 nerve roots.

Cervical facet block. The joint in the cervical spine is located using an X-ray machine, and a local anesthetic and anti-inflammatory are placed in the joint. The local anesthetic works quickly, and if your pain is gone immediately after the procedure, it gives you a diagnostic answer. The steroid can take days to weeks to peak and provide long-term relief. I repeat, if you have pain in the back of the shoulder as well as the arm, I would first start with the cervical nerve root block, as the facet never creates arm pain.

Thoracic nerve root block. The thoracic nerve roots also can create pain in the back of the shoulder either because of a disc herniation or because of foraminal stenosis, which means the narrowing of the hole from which the nerve exits. Any of the thoracic nerve roots from T4 down to T8 can cause pain in the back of the shoulder.

Shoulder block. The shoulder joint can create pain in the back of the shoulder, but usually it creates pain in the front of the shoulder. Whether the pain is in the front or the back of the shoulder, a shoulder block is an easy way to determine whether the pain is coming from the shoulder joint. The shoulder block is a procedure in which a local anesthetic and steroid are placed inside of the shoulder joint. If your pain is gone within thirty minutes after the block, then you know that the pain is coming from the shoulder. This block needs to be done using an X-ray or an ultrasound machine to ensure that the local anesthetic and steroid are actually in the joint. The steroids may take a week or two to kick in and can provide long-term relief.

My Neck Hurts (Chapter 9)

A pain in your neck, if it is coming from your spine, is usually due to an inflamed disc, nerve, or joint in the cervical spine. You may notice that along with the pain, you may have some level of muscle spasm and possibly even headaches. Because the pain from the facets and nerves can be so similar, and the areas in which an inflamed nerve and joint can create pain overlap, it may take several diagnostic procedures to pin down your problem. It is important to do this because your therapy, exercise, and daily activities may be different depending on which structure is creating your pain. Read Chapter 9 for more information on neck pain.

Cervical nerve root block. This procedure is the exact same procedure as a lumbar nerve root block, but in the cervical spine instead. The nerve is treated with a local anesthetic and a steroid anti-inflammatory medication and then assessed immediately afterward for relief. If the pain is gone, you have an answer to what is creating the pain. The steroids may take up to a couple of weeks to completely take effect and offer you long-term relief. The cervical nerves C2, C3, C4, C5, C6, C7, and C8 can all create neck pain. I use patient history, along with the MRI, to determine which specific cervical nerve I will treat to provide a diagnosis as well as to give therapeutic relief.

Cervical facet block. Each cervical facet has a specific area of the neck that it covers, and when inflamed, any of the cervical facets can create neck pain. The joint in the cervical spine is located using an X-ray machine, and a local anesthetic and anti-inflammatory are placed in the joint. The local anesthetic works very quickly, and if the pain is gone immediately after the procedure, it gives a diagnostic answer. The steroid can take days to weeks to peak and can provide long-term relief.

My Arm Hurts—It Tingles and My Fingers Go Numb (Chapter 10)

The usual reason for arm pain, if it is coming from the cervical spine, is that one of the nerves in the cervical spine is inflamed. The nerve can become irritated because of a herniated disc, or inflamed because of the narrowing of the hole from which the nerve exits. You may notice that you have shoulder pain, neck pain, or headaches along with the arm pain. At times, you may only have one of these symptoms; at others, you may have all of them. For example, you may notice that part of your arm hurts one day, and another day, your shoulder may hurt but you don't have arm pain. Of course, you could have that miserable day when your shoulder and arm both hurt and you also have severe neck pain with headaches. The most common cervical nerves that create arm pain are C5, C6, C7, and C8. Chapter 10 provides more information regarding arm pain.

Cervical nerve root block. This procedure is the exact same procedure as a lumbar nerve root block, but in the cervical spine instead. The nerve is treated with a local anesthetic and a steroid anti-inflammatory medication and then assessed immediately afterward for relief. If the pain is gone, you know what is creating the pain. The effect of the steroids may take up to a couple of weeks to completely kick in and provide long-term relief. The pain usually is coming from only one of the nerves in the cervical spine. I may block several nerves on the same day to locate the exact nerve that is creating the pain. If I block one of the nerves and the arm pain is not gone, then I move on to the next nerve until I find the exact cause of the pain.

My Mid-Back Hurts—I Feel Like I Pulled a Muscle (Chapter 11)

The thoracic area is the middle of the spine between the cervical and lumbar areas. The thoracic spine, even though it is protected by the ribs and therefore has less movement, is an area that I commonly treat. The usual bending forward position that you assume in everyday life, such as when you sit for long periods, brush your teeth, and pick things up, can irritate the disc or nerve in the thoracic area. Each nerve in the thoracic area is attached to the bottom of a rib, and therefore you may notice that the pain wraps around the chest. A lot of patients tell me that they feel like they pulled a muscle in their mid-back, but the pain does not go away. Read Chapter 11 for more information regarding thoracic pain.

Thoracic nerve root block. The thoracic nerves cover the entire middle back as seen in Picture 84. These nerves, when inflamed, can create pain that wraps around to the front of your body, or they may just cause pain in your mid-back, from the top of the shoulder down to the back. This procedure is much like the nerve root blocks that are done for the cervical and lumbar spine. This technique enables me to find the exact nerve that is inflamed because of a disc herniation or because of the narrowing of the hole through which the nerve exits. The nerve in the thoracic spine is located using an X-ray machine, and a local anesthetic and anti-inflammatory are placed on the nerve. The local anesthetic works quickly, and if the pain is gone immediately after the procedure, it provides a diagnostic answer. The steroid will take days to weeks to peak and can provide long-term relief.

Thoracic intradiscal steroid injection. This procedure involves placing the local anesthetic and anti-inflammatory *inside* the disc. I do this procedure when there is a tear *inside* the disc, as placing steroids on the *outside* of the disc with a nerve root block is not going to get the job done.

Thoracic facet block. The joint in the thoracic spine can create significant pain anywhere in the mid-back area. The joints never create pain wrapping around the ribs, because the nerve is the only structure that can cause that type of pain when inflamed. The thoracic facets create more pain when you are either standing up in one place or sleeping on your back, because these joints press on each other when your spine is in a straight position. The facet joints are located using an X-ray machine, and a local anesthetic and anti-inflammatory are placed in the joint. The local anesthetic works very quickly, and if the pain is gone immediately after the procedure, it provides a diagnostic answer. The steroids may take days to weeks to peak and can give you long-term relief.

My Pain Is in My Buttock (Chapter 12)

The most common reason for buttock pain is due to the inflammation of one of the structures of the lumbar spine. As discussed in Chapter 12, the usual cause of buttock pain is due to spinal stenosis or one of the lower lumbar discs irritating one of the lumbar nerves. The most common lumbar nerve roots that create pain in the buttock are the L2, L3, L4, L5, and S1 nerve roots. The hip joint, which is located in the groin and not the buttock area, is not a common cause of buttock pain. I consider the hip as a possible source of pain if the patient has groin pain or pain only in the very low part of the buttock. The sacroiliac joint is also not a common cause of buttock pain.

Epidural steroid injection. This is one procedure that is not diagnostic, but it may be therapeutic. An epidural steroid injection is probably the best procedure to relieve pain in the buttock if the lumbar nerves are inflamed because of central spinal stenosis. The epidural attempts to remove the inflammation in the area of the spinal canal that is narrowed. The narrowing can occur at any level, so the combination of the clinical findings and the MRI will help determine which areas need to be treated with the epidural. I usually do an epidural above and below the area of stenosis to try to get the steroids through the area that is narrowed. This procedure needs to be done with an X-ray machine to ensure that you get coverage of the epidural space that is narrowed. If you have had lower back surgery, I recommend that you have a lumbar nerve root block to treat the spinal stenosis, as the epidural space after lumbar surgery may not be intact.

Lumbar nerve root block. A disc herniation or foraminal stenosis at most of the levels of the lumbar spine can create an inflammation of the lumbar nerves and give you buttock pain. The most common lumbar nerve roots that create pain in the buttock are the L2, L3, L4, L5, and S1 nerve roots. The lumbar nerve root block is done to isolate the nerve that is creating the buttock pain and to provide relief by eliminating the inflammation.

Lumbar facet block. The lower lumbar facets at L4-L5 and L5-S1 may create pain in the buttock. The lumbar facet block has to be done using an X-ray machine. A local anesthetic and steroid are placed inside the facet joint, and if the lumbar facet is creating the pain, the pain will be significantly better immediately after the procedure. The steroid that is placed in the lumbar facets, which may take several weeks to take effect, provides long-term relief.

Sacroiliac joint block. The sacroiliac joint is *not* a common cause of buttock pain, even though patients often are given this diagnosis. This procedure has to be done using an X-ray machine, because that is the only way to ensure that the local anesthetic and steroid actually get into the joint. The buttock pain should be gone immediately after placement of the local anesthetic inside the sacroiliac joint, if that is the source of the pain.

Piriformis muscle injection. The piriformis is another very unusual reason patients have buttock pain, but this is another favorite diagnosis given to patients, merely because the piriformis muscle is in the area of the buttock. I consider this procedure only if another cause of buttock pain cannot be identified. This procedure should be done only using ultrasound or an X-ray machine. I use a CT scan to do this block so that I can see the muscle.

My Tailbone Hurts When I Sit (Chapter 13)

The most common causes of pain in the tailbone area usually are the result of irritation of the bone that makes up the coccyx, commonly referred to as the tailbone, or an inflammation of the Ganglion of Impar, which is a set of nerves right below the coccyx. The patient may have tailbone pain if the lumbar nerve root that goes to the area of the tailbone is inflamed. Chapter 13 provides information regarding tailbone pain.

Ganglion of Impar block. This procedure involves finding the set of the nerves under the tailbone, called the Ganglion of Impar, and placing a local anesthetic and a steroidal anti-inflammatory medication on these nerves. This procedure has to be done using an X-ray machine. If these nerves are creating the pain, relief should be immediate following this procedure. The effect of the steroid anti-inflammatory, which may take a couple of weeks to kick in, will provide long-term relief.

Lumbar nerve root block. A disc herniation or foraminal stenosis at the lower levels of the lumbar spine can inflame the nerves in the lumbar spine that cover the area of the tailbone. This procedure isolates the nerve that is creating the tailbone pain and provides some relief by eliminating the inflammation. If the nerve in question is blocked and the pain is coming from the lumbar nerve roots, you should notice immediate relief and be able to sit on the tailbone.

My Groin Hurts (Chapter 14)

Groin pain, if it is caused by an orthopedic or musculoskeletal problem, is usually due to the hip joint or one of the lumbar nerve roots. All the lumbar nerve roots can create groin pain. Thoracic nerves T11 and T12 also can create pain into the groin. Chapter 14 goes into detail regarding groin pain.

Hip block. The hip joint commonly creates pain in the groin when it is inflamed. If the pain is coming from the hip, a diagnostic block of the hip joint will eliminate the groin pain. This procedure should be done using X-ray guidance to ensure that the local anesthetic and steroid mixture actually reaches the hip joint. If the pain is coming from the hip joint, you should notice that the groin pain is gone immediately after the hip joint block. If you still notice pain in the area of the groin, then it tells you that something other than the hip joint is creating the groin pain.

Lumbar nerve root block. Most of the lumbar nerve roots, including L1, L2, L3, L4, L5, and S1, can create groin pain. A lumbar nerve root block will isolate the nerve that is creating the groin pain and provide relief by eliminating the inflammation.

SPINAL DIAGNOSTIC APPROACH VERSUS PAIN MANAGEMENT PROCEDURES

Many patients ask me the difference between taking a spinal diagnostic approach using minimally invasive procedures versus pain management–type care. The answer has to do with two words: *location* and *endpoint*. The idea is that if you can locate the specific problem that is creating your pain, you may be able to reach an endpoint with your pain. That endpoint may be that your pain goes away, or it may even be surgery. But there is an endpoint.

> **Remember: You have to find the exact location that is creating your pain to be able to diagnose what is creating your pain.** *Diagnose and then treat.*
>
> **If you cannot diagnose the problem that is creating your pain, you cannot treat it to reach an endpoint. If you cannot at least try and reach an endpoint, you are looking at long-term pain management, meaning pain management procedures and possible narcotics.**

Let me give you a few examples of pain management injections versus minimally invasive diagnostic procedures.

The most common type of injection that has been used for "pain management" is the epidural steroid injection or caudal epidural steroid injection. I discussed this procedure earlier in this chapter, but basically it is a procedure that involves placing steroids and local anesthetic in the epidural space. This procedure is done in the pain management setting both with and without using an X-ray machine to guide the placement. This is a non-specific procedure that is based on the hope that the spread of local anesthetic and steroids may reach the inflamed structure in the spine. If you do not get relief from the epidural, or even if you get short-term relief and your pain returns, you are back to the starting point. You still do not know the exact structure that is creating your pain.

By using a diagnostic minimally invasive procedure, either a nerve root block, a selective facet block, or an intradiscal injection, you can pin down the location of your problem. If you do not get long-term relief, you can consider a surgical option to try and fix the issue. There is another reason why you want to locate the exact problem. I will talk about this in the next chapter, but depending on the exact structure that is creating your pain, the therapy, exercises, and body mechanics will be different. If you have pain due to an inflamed facet, the way you move, sleep, and exercise will be different than if your discomfort is caused by an irritated disc. If you use the same therapy and exercises for facet problems as you do for disc issues, you are going to make your pain worse! You need to know what is creating your pain so that you will know how not to re-aggravate your problem.

Trigger point injections are another procedure done frequently by medical practitioners for pain management. This technique was first performed at a time when we did not know that certain structures in the spine created specific types of pain. We would just stick a needle into the muscle to break up the spasm or inject steroids into areas of the body where patients said they had pain. Trigger point injections can be done just with a needle without using any medications, which is called dry needling, or the injection can be done using steroids and a local anesthetic. We now know that most muscle spasms because of spine pain are actually due to one of the structures in the spine being inflamed, as each structure has nerves that go to the muscles. So when one of the nerves, discs, or facets is inflamed, it sends a signal to the muscle, which in turn creates the spasm. If you treat the actual cause of the muscle spasm, which is the structure in the spine, you will eliminate the muscle spasm without sticking needles in the muscle.

Is there a place for trigger point injections? Absolutely. If the primary problem is a muscle, as when you pull or traumatize the muscle, then a trigger point injection may help in the healing process. For example, tennis elbow, which is an irritation of the muscle, can be treated with a trigger point injection. Another example would be if you pulled one of your muscles in your back or hamstring muscles while you are twisting or running. There is also a place for trigger point injections in the first several weeks of your spine pain. The trigger point injections may give you relief while your spine is healing. But after the first four to six weeks, you are better off eliminating the actual cause of the muscle spasm by treating the structure in your spine that is creating it, instead of just injecting the muscle; unless you eliminate the original inflammation, the pain and muscle spasm will return. And again, no endpoint!

WHY SOME SPINAL INJECTIONS DO NOT WORK—ALL ABOUT LOCATION, LOCATION, LOCATION

Over the last twenty years I have had numerous patients who have asked me this question—usually because they are still hurting and are not sure what to do next. Why is it that some spinal injections do not work? The answer is all about one thing: *location, location, location.* You have to locate the exact structure that is creating the pain to be able to eliminate the inflammation and eradicate the pain.

The first reason that you are not going to get relief from a spinal procedure is that the procedure never got the steroids to the area that was inflamed.

Let me give you an example. **Picture 116** shows how an epidural steroid injection is placed into an area of spinal stenosis. The idea is to decrease the inflammation and eliminate the pain. This is an appropriate procedure for this problem and may give you good relief.

Picture 117 shows why this same epidural is not effective for a disc herniation creating inflammation around a specific nerve. The steroids placed into the epidural space are *not* anywhere close to the disc herniation that is inflaming the nerve.

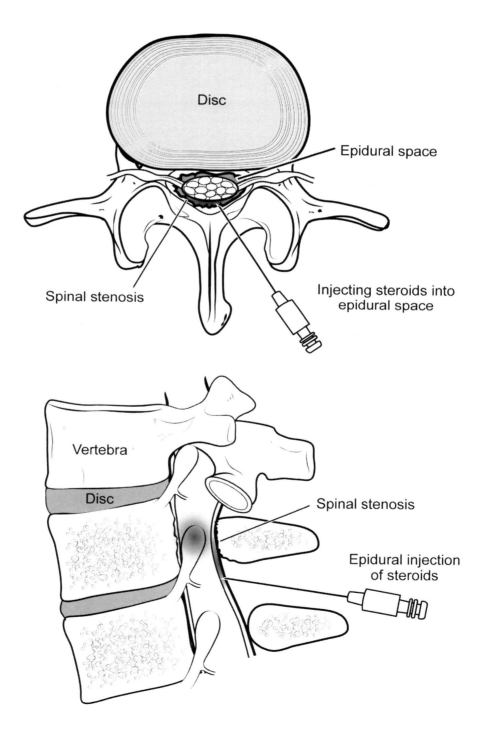

Disc

Epidural space

Spinal stenosis

Injecting steroids into epidural space

Vertebra

Disc

Spinal stenosis

Epidural injection of steroids

PICTURE 116

Epidural steroid injection for spinal stenosis.

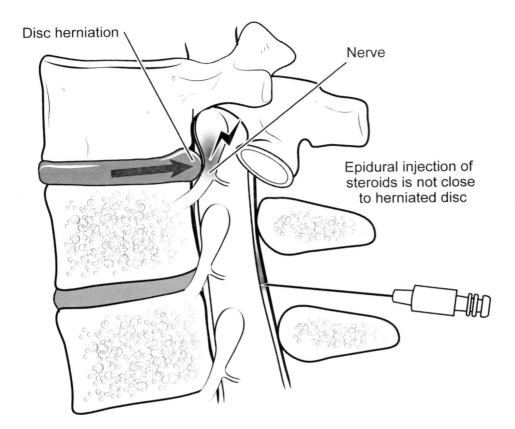

Disc herniation

Nerve

Epidural injection of steroids is not close to herniated disc

PICTURE 117

Failure of epidural steroid injection to reach the nerve that the disc herniation is inflaming.

A patient who has a disc herniation that is inflaming a specific nerve is better served by a procedure called a nerve root injection, which is far superior to the epidural, both diagnostically and therapeutically (**Picture 118**).

If you have a herniated disc inflaming the nerve, or arthritis narrowing the hole through which the nerve exits, there is a better chance that you will get relief because the steroids are being placed directly on top of the nerve. It is *all* about one thing: *location*.

Let me take this example one step further. If you look at Picture 118, you will see a bulging disc at one level and foraminal stenosis at the other. The bulging disc or the foraminal stenosis could create an inflammation of the nerve at either level. If you have a nerve root block performed at the level with the bulging disc, but it is actually the foraminal stenosis at the other level that is creating your pain, you will not get better. So even if you have a nerve root block, if it is not at the level where the inflammation is, you still will not get better. You have to get the medication to the exact right spot. *Location*.

Let me give you another example of why you may have had injections and never had much relief. **Picture 119** illustrates the different parts of the spine and the procedures that should be used depending on which part of the spine is inflamed. The left side of this picture shows the different parts of the spine that could be inflamed and the right side shows which procedure you should have depending on which structure is inflamed.

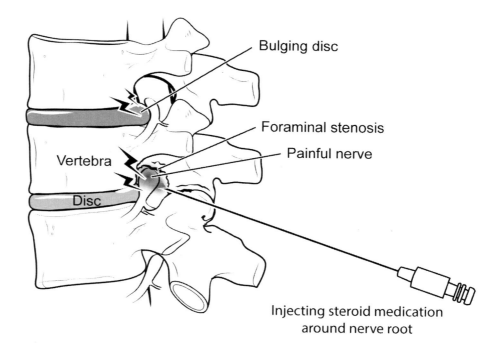

Bulging disc

Foraminal stenosis

Painful nerve

Vertebra

Disc

Injecting steroid medication
around nerve root

Picture 119 shows:

1. If you have an inflamed annular tear *inside* the disc, your best procedure is an intradiscal steroid injection.

2. If you have an inflamed nerve root due to the irritation of the *outside* of the herniated disc, your best procedure is a nerve root block.

3. If you have an inflamed facet joint, your best procedure is a facet block.

Now what happens if you have an inflamed tear inside your disc and your physician performs an epidural? *Absolutely nothing.* Or what happens if the physician performs a facet block even though your pain is coming from the disc herniation inflaming the nerve root? *Absolutely nothing.* What happens if you are having pain going down your arm or leg because of a disc herniation and the physician does an RFTC procedure and burns the nerve to the facets? *Absolutely nothing.*

You have to treat the structure that is inflamed to get pain relief!

The real problem is that if you do not obtain a diagnosis and/or get better, you may be forced to take narcotics to keep your pain under control, which, as you read in Chapter 15, is not the best way to treat spine pain!

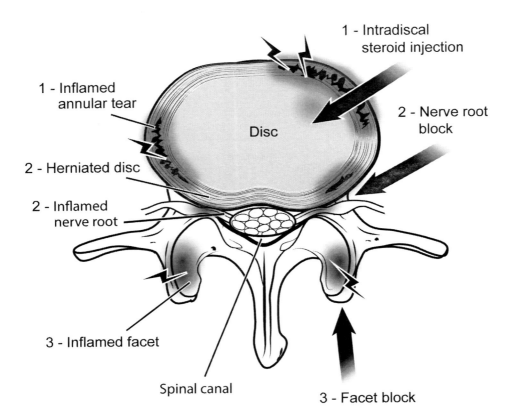

1 - Intradiscal steroid injection

1 - Inflamed annular tear

Disc

2 - Nerve root block

2 - Herniated disc

2 - Inflamed nerve root

3 - Inflamed facet

Spinal canal

3 - Facet block

PICTURE 119

Inflamed parts of the spine and the procedure used for each area.

SUMMARY

1. This chapter provides a rundown of minimally invasive procedures that can be performed to correctly diagnose the source of pain and, in some cases, to provide therapeutic benefits.

2. The goal is to diagnose the problem, eliminate the inflammation, and provide long-term relief.

3. All procedures should be done using an X-ray machine and all pictures of the procedures must be saved. This will ensure that you are getting the correct procedure and that the anti-inflammatory steroid actually got to the structure that was inflamed.

4. What separates this approach from chronic pain management? The procedures that usually are done in pain management clinics do not attempt to diagnose the problem or to find a long-term solution for the problem. These procedures usually are combined with long-term usage of narcotic medications.

5. The common procedures that are used primarily for chronic pain management are epidural steroid injections, non-diagnostic facet blocks, burning of the nerves to the facets, and trigger point injections.

6. The use of central epidural steroid injections has no place in a spinal diagnostic approach, as no diagnostic information can be derived from it.

7. The only appropriate use of the epidural is as a therapeutic maneuver for patients who have central spinal stenosis.

8. The steroid from any of the injections takes several weeks to peak, and therefore the procedure should not be repeated until the full effect of the first injection is realized.

9. If you still have discomfort several weeks after the first procedure, a second procedure is warranted.

10. Do not undergo any more procedures if you are pain-free after the first injection. These procedures work by eliminating inflammation, and if you are having *no* pain, there is no inflammation for the steroids to work on.

11. Diagnostic and therapeutic injections of the spine will not work if the steroid does not get to the area that is inflamed, or if the right procedure is not used for the specific structure that is inflamed.

12. Identify the specific structure that is creating the pain and eliminate the inflammation in that structure.

13. Once that has been accomplished, the next step is to change your body mechanics and lifestyle so that the structure, whether it is the disc, joint, or nerve, does not continue to become re-inflamed.

14. If the minimally invasive approach fails, you will still know the exact structure that is creating your pain so that you can consider a surgical approach.

15. The idea is to have an endpoint and *not* to create chronic pain!

The *Straight Spine Safe Spine* Therapy and Exercise Program

INTRODUCTION TO THE *STRAIGHT SPINE SAFE SPINE* PROGRAM

The primary reason you get better after having spine pain is because the body heals itself in the first four to six weeks, not because you do any specific exercise. There are only a few exercises that are currently being used in therapy that really do anything to help resolve your pain, and some of them will actually create more pain, if they are not specific to the problem that is creating your pain. I will talk about this a little later in the chapter.

What is more important than specific exercises that may help you decrease your pain is to avoid aggravating your spine while it is healing. You can do that by using proper body posture and mechanics and learning how to strengthen your arms, legs, and abdominal muscles without aggravating the problem in your spine.

The **Straight Spine Safe Spine**™ Program is an exercise and body mechanics program that is designed for those of you who either are currently in pain or have had your pain recently resolved. This program is unique in that it combines three important parts into one "therapy" program:

1. It teaches you how to use proper body posture and mechanics, which will allow the problem in your spine to heal and keep you from re-aggravating the *specific* problem in your spine.

2. It gives you exercises that will help you feel better while your body heals itself, while not aggravating the *specific* problem in your spine. Your spine should be *straight* for most of these exercises.

3. It shows you how to strengthen your body in a *safe* way, while not aggravating the *specific* problem in your spine, by teaching you how to exercise while keeping your spine *straight*.

Can you tell that I want the spine *straight* while you do therapy, exercises, and your daily activities, and I want you to do things *safely* so that you can let the spine heal and not re-aggravate it after you are feeling better?

The **Straight Spine Safe Spine** Program will teach you exercises that are *specific* for your problem. Most of the physical therapy exercises that are currently used for spine pain are not *specific* for the problem that may be creating your pain. For example, your back pain may be due to a herniated disc, arthritic joints in your spine, or spinal stenosis. Some of the exercises currently used in physical therapy are excellent for the acute herniated disc, because they help move the disc away from the nerve and reduce the pain going down the leg. For example, lying on the floor and arching your back is a good exercise if a herniated disc is creating your leg pain (**Picture 120**).

But, if you have spinal stenosis or if your pain is coming from the facet joints in the back of your spine, you are going to *aggravate* your condition by doing the exercise in Picture 120. The arching of your back will either close down the canal with spinal stenosis or irritate the facets in the back of your spine. The patient with spinal stenosis or facet pain may have pain in the same area of the body as someone with a herniated disc, but will need a *different* exercise than the patient with a herniated disc.

Another example of the wrong exercise for the problem is if you have pain and spasm in your hamstring muscle because of an inflamed lumbar nerve in your back. The exercise in **Picture 121**, which basically stretches the hamstring, is a common exercise used by trainers and therapists if you have a problem with your hamstring and you need it stretched out.

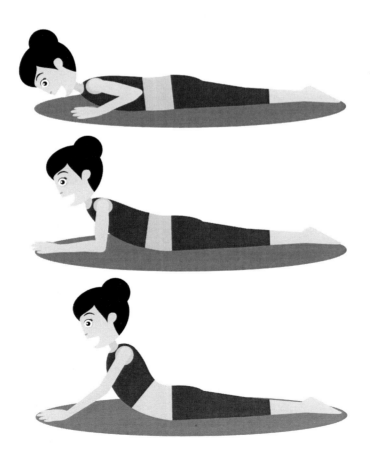

PICTURE 120

Exercise that may help push the herniated disc away from the nerve.

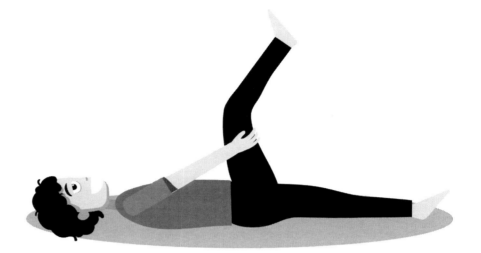

Stretching the hamstring, but pulling on the lumbar nerve roots.

But, if your hamstring is tight because of an inflamed lumbar nerve due to a disc herniation, then stretching your leg, as shown in Picture 121, is going to actually pull on your lumbar (sciatic) nerves. And guess what? Because the lumbar nerves are connected to the hamstring muscles, irritating your inflamed lumbar (sciatic) nerve is going to cause the hamstring muscles to tighten up even more. The patient with pain and tightness in the hamstring muscles because of an inflamed lumbar nerve root needs a *different* exercise than someone who has a tight hamstring because of a muscle problem.

Another example is when patients with back and leg pain are told to start on a regular walking program, because this form of exercise will strengthen the legs. That will definitely help patients with a herniated disc who feel better when they walk, but if your back and leg pain is caused by spinal stenosis, which is a narrowing of your spinal canal, and you walk a lot, you actually will aggravate your underlying problem. The patient with spinal stenosis needs a *different* way to exercise, one that is specific for spinal stenosis.

The **Straight Spine Safe Spine** Program teaches you proper body mechanics so that you do *not* re-aggravate the *specific* problem in your spine. The length of relief after your inflammation and pain go away primarily depends on how long you can keep the herniated disc, nerve, or facet joint from becoming re-inflamed—no matter how degenerated your spine is. The key is to exercise and strengthen your muscles so that you can use proper body mechanics in your daily activities to avoid re-aggravating your spine. Body mechanics involve two things: (1) the position of your body when you are not moving, such as sitting or sleeping, and (2) the way you move your body when you are active, such as picking up a box or emptying your dishwasher. If you know the *specific* problem in your spine, it will help you decide on the right body positions and body movements.

The position of your body, even when it is not moving, can create problems in your spine. For example, sitting creates more pressure on your discs than when you are standing. So if you just got over a painful disc problem with your back or neck and then go back to sitting a lot at work, your pain may come back as the disc becomes inflamed again. If you have spinal stenosis and you stand a lot, this position is going to make your stenosis pain worse.

How you move your body also plays a role in possibly re-inflaming the structures of the spine. For example, let us say you have a lumbar disc herniation that creates pain down the leg or a cervical disc herniation that creates neck pain, and you pick up a box without bending your knees. As the body bends forward, while keeping the legs straight, pressure is increased on *all* the discs in the spine, which in turn may create inflammation (**Picture 122**).

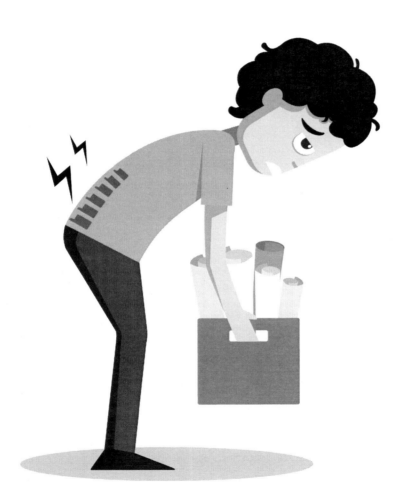

PICTURE 122

Picking up a box with your back instead of your legs.

Now let's look at the same maneuver if you pick up the box by bending the knees and keeping the lower back straight (**Picture 123**).

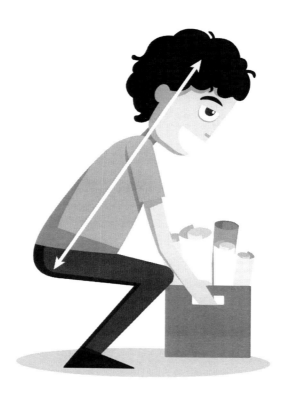

PICTURE 123

Picking up a box with your legs.

When you bend your knees and keep your spine straight, the disc has less pressure placed on it, which in turn decreases the possibility of the disc pushing against the nerve. This is just one example, but bending your back without bending your knees is a common movement that you use every day: emptying the dishwasher, taking clothes out of the washing machine, brushing your teeth, working in the yard, taking things out of the car, putting on your shoes, reaching for things on the floor or under the counter. As you see, you have the chance to bend wrong all day long. This increased pressure that you place on the discs and the nerves by using the wrong body mechanics will at some point aggravate these structures and put you back into pain by creating inflammation around the disc and the nerve.

This concept does not apply just to the disc and nerve. Let's say that you know that your pain is coming from the facet joints in the back of your spine. Exercises that commonly are given for sciatic pain, which involves arching your back repeatedly, would make your pain worse. Swimming, which is a great exercise for someone with a herniated disc, may aggravate your spine while it is in an arched position when you swim. You would be better off walking in a pool instead of swimming so that your facets do not become re-inflamed. Doing yoga, which also involves movements in which you arch your spine, can aggravate your facets. These examples demonstrate why you need to know exactly what is creating your pain before you start to exercise.

SPECIFIC BODY POSTURE, BODY MECHANICS, AND EXERCISES FOR EACH PART OF THE SPINE

The **Straight Spine Safe Spine** Program is a complete therapy and exercise program that is designed to show you how to use proper body mechanics and posture so that you do not re-aggravate the *specific* structure causing your pain, and at the same time teach you exercises that may decrease your pain as well as safely strengthen your body so that you will quit placing stress on your spine.

The rest of this chapter is divided into the cervical, thoracic, and lumbar areas of the spine. For example, if you have a problem in your lumbar spine, you will notice that in the lumbar section I cover the correct body posture and body mechanics that will allow your spine to heal and keep you from having recurrences of pain, as well as give you specific exercises you should do or *not* do depending on whether your pain results from a disc herniation, facet inflammation, or spinal stenosis. How do you decide which structure is creating your pain? By reading the first several chapters of this book as well as the chapter in Part II that most closely resembles your pain. You can also ask your therapist or physician for guidance.

What sets **Straight Spine Safe Spine** apart from most spine therapy programs is the *specific* exercises for the *specific* problem. An exercise that may be very helpful for someone with a disc herniation may actually make your pain worse if you have spinal stenosis. I am also going to give you information on how to continue to exercise and strengthen your muscles without aggravating the *specific* structure in your spine that was creating your problem. For example, if you just got over having neck and arm pain because of a cervical disc herniation in your neck, how can you still exercise your abdominals without aggravating your neck?

I do not want to complicate matters, but you may have decided after reading the earlier chapters in this book that your pain may be coming from different sources. You may have leg pain from a disc herniation as well as back pain from facets. I recommend that you read both the lumbar disc herniation section as well as the lumbar facet section. There are two things that I stress in this chapter. The first is that most of the exercises for the spine involve very little movement of the spine, and therefore you can use most of them to help you strengthen your body no matter what your problem is. The second is if an exercise creates pain, don't do it! The body is telling you that you may be aggravating your problem.

The last thing I should remind you of is that most of the time your pain is going to go away if you can keep from aggravating the problem that is creating your pain—not because of a specific exercise. Do not get wrapped up in specific exercises as a source of relief. Instead, look at this program as a learning process for you and the rest of your body so that you will not continue to have episodes of spine pain!

Cervical Spine

CERVICAL SPINE BODY POSTURE AND MECHANICS

Cervical disc and nerve

If you have a problem with a disc herniation in your cervical spine and you have had neck, shoulder, or arm pain, you first have to remember where the disc sits. The disc sits in the *front* of the spine, and when you bend your head down, you increase the pressure in the disc. This may not create any issues in a young person's spine, but **Picture 124** illustrates a normally aging spine with herniated discs and bone spurs.

Chronic bad posture with the head bent down all day, a position common for people looking at computers and cellular phones, can lead to inflamed discs. If the disc is inflamed, it may lead to increased neck pain. This inflammation is becoming so common that the problem is now called "text neck."

Picture 125 shows in the top image that the basic head position should be looking straight ahead with no bending or twisting of the neck.

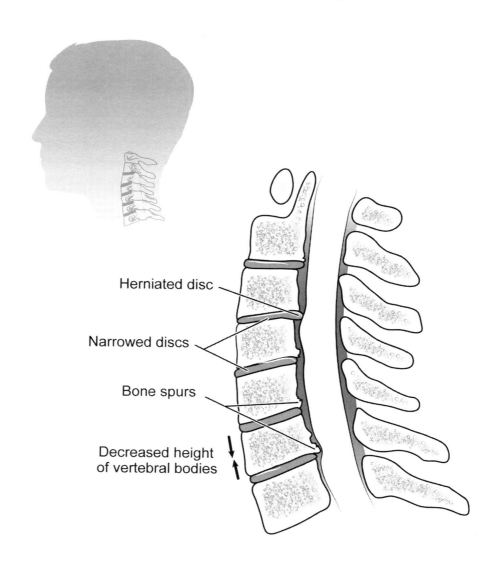

Herniated disc

Narrowed discs

Bone spurs

Decreased height
of vertebral bodies

PICTURE 124

Spine with herniated
discs and bone spurs.

Best head position is straight

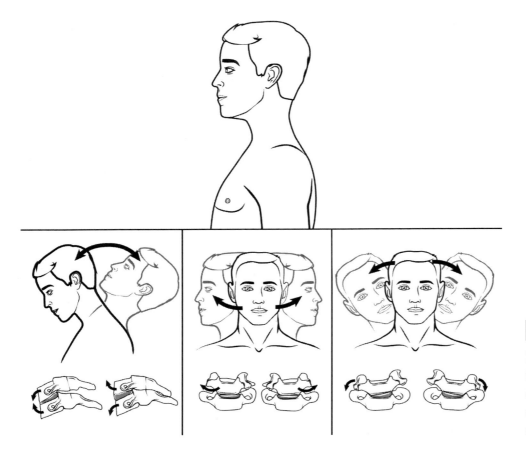

PICTURE 125

Bending your head forward and rotating or twisting your neck can aggravate your discs.

The three lower images in Picture 125 show that increased stress is placed on the discs no matter how you move your head, whether up and down, rotated side to side, or bent side to side. The first image on the left shows that as you bend your head forward, the disc in the neck becomes compressed. The image also shows that when you arch your neck backward, the bones separate and the disc has more space, but you then will put stress on your facet joints. The middle image shows that as you rotate your neck to either side, the bones in your neck will rotate, which will create a twisting motion of the disc. The image on the right shows that as you bend your head to either side, the sides of the disc are compressed. Therefore, the perfect position of the neck for anyone, even if you never have had neck pain, is to keep your head up and back over your shoulders at all times with little twisting, turning, or bending of your neck!

The way you hold your head and move your neck on a daily basis is more important than all the exercises! If I can tell you one simple thing to remember, it would be to always keep your spine straight and try not to move your neck. If you bend down to pick something up, make sure that you bend your knees and keep your head over your shoulders. This means when you empty the dishwasher, take clothes out of the washing machine, wash your face, and even make the bed (**Picture 126**).

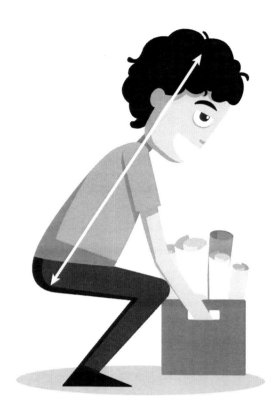

Keeping your head over the top of your shoulders.

The more careful you are about not moving your neck out of the neutral position, the less irritation of the structures in the neck. Many times, you may not even be moving your body, but you are creating pressure on your discs just by sitting at a desk, reading a book, looking at a computer, driving a car, watching television in bed, and looking at your cell phone. All these activities involve looking down or twisting your neck, even though you are not moving the rest of your body. You cannot stop all movement of the neck, but the more you remember this neutral position, the more you will change how you do things. You should prop the book up when you read, elevate the computer on your desk so that your head stays up **(Picture 127)**, sit up in bed to watch television, look up frequently if you are sitting at a desk, keep your head back against the headrest while you are driving, and learn to turn your body to talk to people instead of just twisting your neck.

The best position for your neck, as well as your whole spine, is when you are standing, because this will keep your spine completely aligned. Standing is actually better than sitting straight up in a chair, because we all have the tendency to tilt the head forward when sitting. When you are standing, the head naturally tends to stay back over the shoulders. I encourage patients to use a sit-stand desk, which will allow you to move the desk up and down **(Picture 128)**.

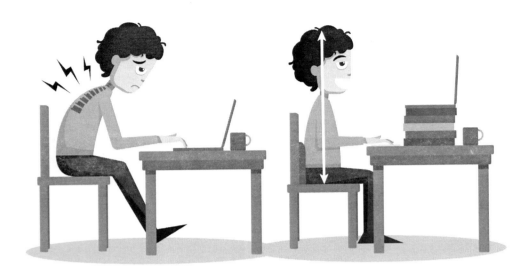

Sitting in a neutral, head-over-the-shoulder position.

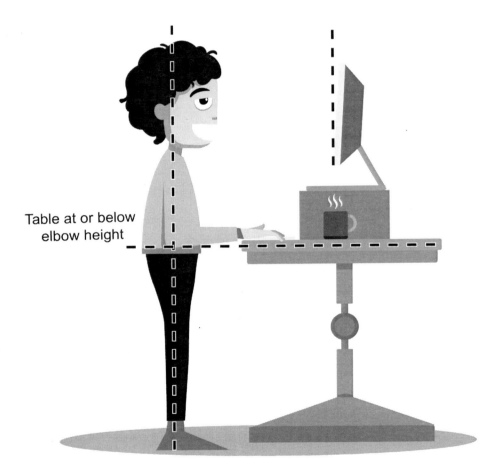

Table at or below elbow height

PICTURE 128

Sit-stand desk.

You should also position your neck in a neutral position while you sleep. Whether you lie on your back or on your side, use a pillow that keeps your neck in a neutral position **(Picture 129)**. This is usually a fairly thin, flat pillow.

Do not sleep on your stomach. Doing so forces you to turn your head in one direction and possibly puts more pressure on the disc and nerve. If you

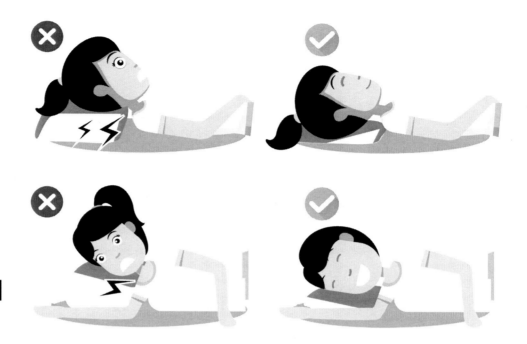

PICTURE 129

Sleeping with your head in a neutral position.

are hurting, you should sleep in whichever position makes your neck feel better. Depending on the placement of the disc and how inflamed it is, you may have to sleep partially sitting up until the pain starts to subside. Or with your arm over your head.

Cervical facets

If your pain is coming from your cervical facet joints, the first thing you should know is that the facets are located in the back of the spine, which is exactly opposite of the discs (**Picture 130**).

The facets move away from each other as you bend your head down and press on each other as you bend your head backward (**Picture 131**).

Bending your head forward will take the pressure off the facets, which is the exact opposite of the discs. Rotation or bending your neck to the sides can aggravate the cervical facets.

The positions, postures, and ways to move your body if you have problems with your cervical facets are very similar to those described for patients with cervical disc and nerve pain except for a few things that I want to mention. Therefore, I suggest you read the above section on body posture and mechanics for the disc and nerve first and then read the rest of this section. An important difference between facets and discs is that if you have a problem with your cervical facets, you should try to keep from arching your neck, as you may aggravate your facets, which are located in the back of the

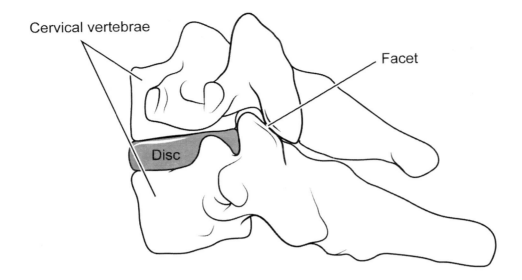

Cervical vertebrae

Facet

Disc

PICTURE 130

Cervical facet in the back of the spine.

spine. For example, if you want to look up at something, you should back up and look from a distance, instead of bending your neck backward. When it comes to the cervical spine, whether it is the disc, nerve, or facet, do *not* move your neck as much as possible. Move your body instead.

Resting for patients with cervical facet pain can be painful, especially if you tend to sleep on your back or on your stomach, because that puts your neck in an extended or rotated position, which creates pressure on your joints. If you have a cervical facet problem, the best position is to sleep on your side, with a pillow that keeps your head in a neutral position, and have your neck curled in a fetal position. This will keep your head bent forward, which will keep the facets from pressing on each other. You can sleep on your back if you really have to, but use a larger pillow that will keep your head bent forward so that the facet joints stay open (**Picture 132**).

The more your neck stays in a neutral position, the less chance there will be of aggravating the facets, the discs, or the nerves. As much as possible, I want you to move the rest of your body instead of your neck for all your activities. Bend your knees and move your feet to keep your head directly over the top of your shoulders.

The basic position of the neck should always be a neutral position over your shoulders, and remember to avoid turning or twisting the neck any more than you have to. I am not a believer in using neck collars or braces to protect your neck because they will weaken your neck muscles, but it may be helpful to use a collar or brace for short periods of time after an episode of neck pain just to remind you to keep your neck straight.

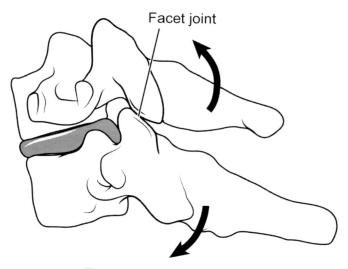

Facet joint

Flexion (bending forward)

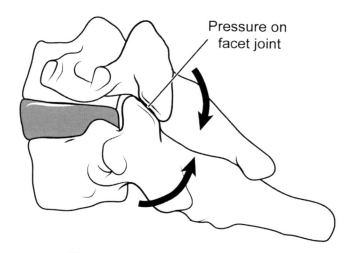

Pressure on facet joint

Extension (bending backward)

PICTURE 131

Facet joints open when you bend your head forward and press on each other when you bend your head backward.

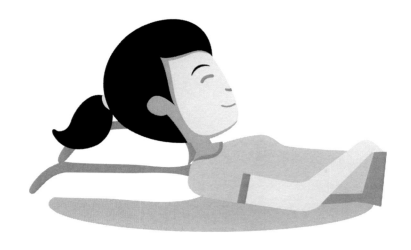

PICTURE 132

Sleeping with your head bent forward to keep your facet joints open.

EXERCISES FOR CERVICAL DISC AND NERVE PAIN

Most therapy programs use twisting and turning exercises of the neck to help the patient strengthen the neck muscles and obtain a greater range of motion. This is the worst thing you can do because it may actually irritate the cervical disc or nerve. Almost every exercise for the cervical spine should involve strengthening the neck muscles without moving the neck! These same exercises can be used whether you are hurting or feeling better, as the same exercises that may help you decrease your pain will also strengthen your neck muscles. These are considered isometric exercises, which are exercises to contract and strengthen the muscle *without moving* the neck. Remember, moving your head up and down or twisting your neck may lead to the disc or nerve becoming inflamed.

Before I talk about isometric exercises for the neck, I want to review one exercise that may be helpful for disc and nerve problems, as it is the only exercise where there is some movement of the neck. This extension exercise is shown in **Picture 133**. Recall the image on the left-hand side of Picture 125, which shows that as you bend your head backward, the disc space opens up. Most patients with disc and nerve pain feel better when they arch their heads backward because the disc space opens up. Slowly go from a neutral position to an arched neck position, and then bring the head back to neutral. Start with three sets of ten neck extensions. I have several disc herniations in my neck, and I do this exercise on a routine basis because it makes my neck feel better *and* it reminds me to keep my head up.

If your neck hurts when you do this exercise, do *not* do it. Depending on the position of the disc herniation, you actually may create more pressure on the disc or nerve. This exercise can create pain if your pain is coming from the facet joints in the back of the neck or if you have spinal stenosis in the neck.

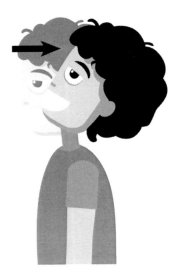

PICTURE 133

Extension exercise of the neck.

> **Remember: Never do exercises that hurt!**

The body is trying to tell you something when it creates pain. Stop! This is one of the reasons that I like isometric exercises, because there is not much movement of the neck with these types of exercises and thus very little chance of aggravating the structures of the neck.

The following exercises for the neck are considered isometric exercises, which strengthen the neck by contracting the muscles with minimal movement of the neck.

To do the chin push-back exercise, shown in **Picture 134**, just push your chin back while your neck is relaxed but keep your head in a neutral position. This repositions your neck over the top of your shoulders while strengthening your neck muscles. Do *not* push the chin down, just back. You can repeat this as many times as you want. The back of your neck should just feel tight as you push back, but not painful. If this exercise hurts, do not do it until you can do it without having pain!

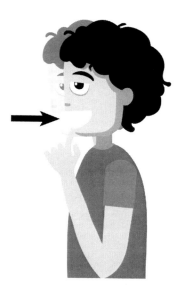

PICTURE 134

Chin push-back exercise.

The next exercise is a standing push-back exercise. While you are standing, push your head back up against a wall for a few seconds and then relax. This will strengthen your neck muscles as well as teach you to keep your head back over your shoulders. This exercise also can be done when sitting by pushing your head back against a headrest of a car seat or the headrest of your office chair (**Picture 135**). Again, remember to keep your head in a neutral position when you do this. There is no limit to how many of these you do. I do this exercise continuously in the car, as I use the headrest to push back against.

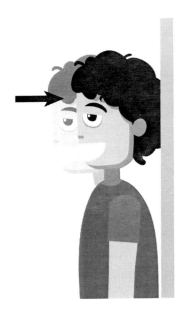

If you don't have a headrest or wall to push your head back against, you can get the same effect by pushing your hands against your head in all four quadrants (front, back, left, right) while your head stays in a neutral position (**Picture 136**). Do this exercise in a standing position. Resist your head against your hand for a few seconds and then relax.

Traction for the neck is a helpful therapeutic modality for patients with disc and nerve pain, because it attempts to give the disc and nerve more room to heal. The two devices that I like for traction of the neck are the Saunders traction machine and the cervical traction collar. The Saunders is used lying down, and the cervical traction collar can be used in any position. I have used both, and they work well. The cervical traction collar, which is more portable, works as a brace to keep your neck straight and also has the capability to provide traction. I take the cervical traction collar on plane flights with me because I can use it as a neck brace, which makes me look straight ahead when I am reading, as well as providing support for my neck in case I fall asleep. If I am hurting, I just pump up the traction on the collar.

The next set of exercises is not specifically for the neck, but for the upper body and abdomen. The way you are going to limit your recurrences of neck pain is by exercising your upper and lower body, including your abdomen, so that you can decrease the stress on the spine. Use the muscles in the rest of your body instead of your spine. If you have had neck pain, the areas of the body that you have to be careful with when you exercise are the upper body and the abdomen. Exercises for the legs should not affect your neck unless you are doing squats with weights on your shoulders. You can find spine-safe exercises for the legs in the lumbar section of this chapter.

Wait to begin these exercises until most of your neck and arm pain is gone. I have lived with herniated discs in my neck for many years but still

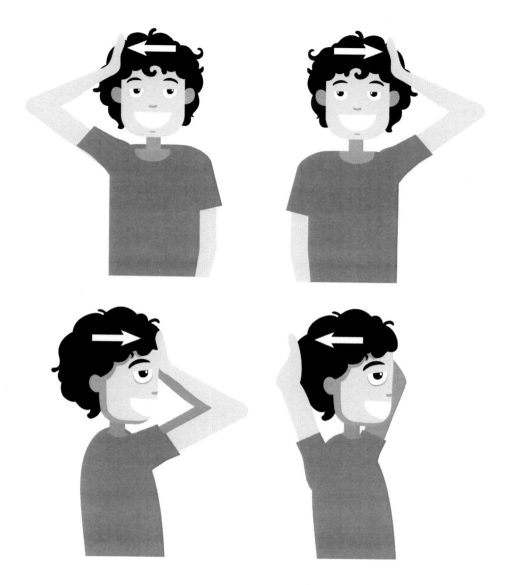

PICTURE 136

Using your hands
to push against
your head.

manage to exercise and lift weights daily. Although I live with a low level of discomfort in my neck that comes and goes, I still work out with no additional aggravation.

Always use light enough weight so that you can avoid moving or jerking your neck. We now know that you can build the same muscle strength by using less weight but doing a higher number of repetitions. I do three sets with each exercise and do fifteen repetitions. One way to keep your head from moving is to do most of your weight lifting on machines, because this will stabilize the weights and keep the stress off your neck. Remember to keep your head from moving and ensure that your head stays back over your shoulders. For example, if you are going to do a common exercise called a pull-down, stand up to grab the bar instead of reaching for it before you sit back down, and pull the bar down in front of your neck instead of behind the neck **(Picture 137)**. Make sure your palms are facing you because that will take some of the stress off your neck, and use light enough weight so that there is no jerking of your neck.

Another example of an exercise to build upper-body strength is a back row as shown in **Picture 138**. I would point out to you that you have to keep your neck over your shoulders and your spine straight when you are doing this exercise.

Keeping your arms strong is very important if you have had problems with neck pain, no matter whether it is due to the disc, nerve, or facet joint. This involves strengthening your triceps and biceps muscles. You want to keep your neck straight when you are exercising your triceps. I usually use a pulley form of machine to exercise my triceps **(Picture 139)**.

As you can see in Picture 139, the head stays over the top of the shoulders and the arms are locked to your side so that it is difficult to move your neck while you pull the bar down.

I recommend using free weights when working on your biceps if you have had a problem with your neck. Most bicep machines are used while you are sitting, and they also make you reach forward to grab the handles of the machine. This position is going to make you move your neck forward and will not allow you to keep your head over your shoulders. By standing and locking your arms by your side and then doing bicep curls, you will keep your head back over your shoulders **(Picture 140)**. And the standing position is a lot better for your neck than sitting.

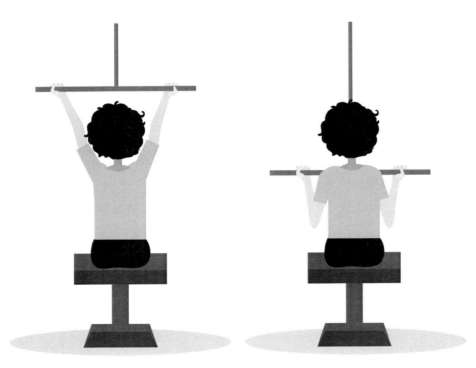

PICTURE 137

Back pull-downs with palms facing you.

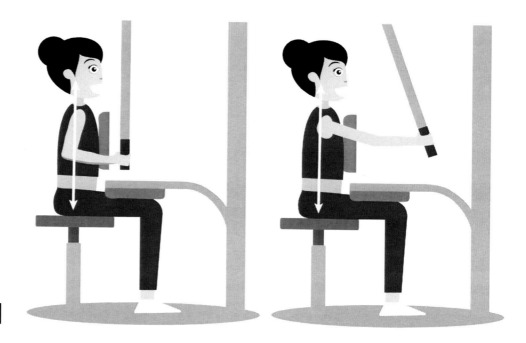

PICTURE 138

Back rows.

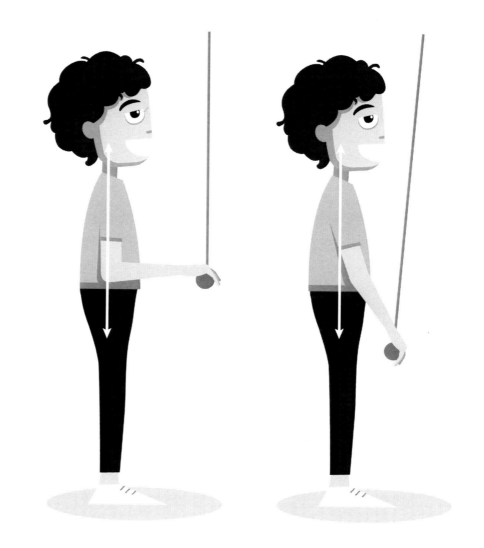

PICTURE 139

Tricep pushdowns.

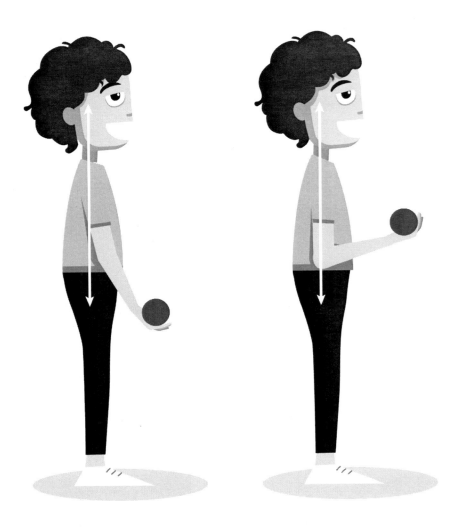

Bicep curls.

You should also *not* allow your head to hang over your neck even if your neck is straight while exercising. Two examples of this are pushups or planks, both of which would put a lot of stress on your neck, because your neck has to try to hold the weight of your head while you are doing these types of exercises. Another example is doing a chest press using dumbbells on a bench instead of a machine. Your neck is going to have to hold the weight of your head as you go through the motion of positioning yourself on the bench. I use a chest press machine instead of doing pushups or using free weights to strengthen my arms and chest (**Picture 141**). I roll up a towel and place it behind my neck when I am using the chest press machine as it helps stabilize my neck, and if the towel falls out, I know that I moved my neck.

Be careful with sit-ups or crunches as the movement can aggravate your neck. You can do the following two exercises instead of sit-ups, as they will strengthen your abdominal muscles without moving your neck. The first one is an isometric abdominal muscle contraction (**Picture 142**). You can sit, stand, or lie down to do this exercise. You place your hand over your

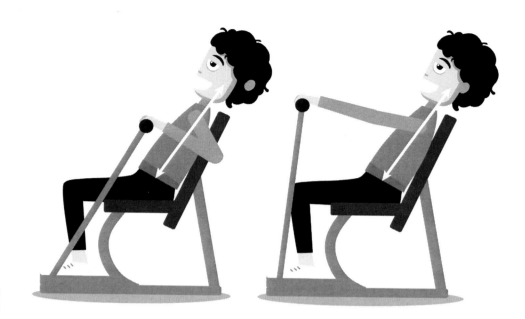

PICTURE 141

Chest press.

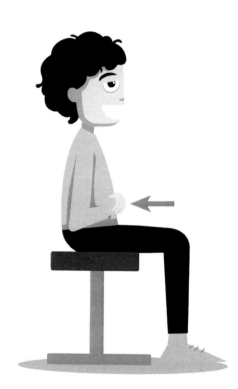

PICTURE 142

Isometric abdominal
muscle contraction.

stomach muscles and then contract your stomach muscles. Hold for five seconds and then relax. You can do as many as you want. Once you get used to doing this exercise you do not need to keep your hands over your stomach muscles. I just want to make sure you feel your muscles contracting when you first start to do this exercise. I do this exercise all day long, whether I am driving in the car or standing in one place.

The next stomach exercise shown in **(Picture 143)** is a sitting abdominal crunch. Keep your spine straight and bring your knees up toward your chest as you contract your stomach muscles. Hold for a couple of seconds and then bring your legs back down, but do not allow them to touch the floor. Repeat. Start with a set of ten and as your stomach muscles become stronger you can increase the number of repetitions.

If you have neck pain, I recommend doing aerobic exercises which are low-impact, using an exercise bike, elliptical trainer, or a StairMaster. I do not advocate running because that is going to create a pounding of your neck structures, but I have a lot of patients who go back to running and have minimal problems with recurrences of their neck pain. If you notice that your pain continues to reoccur when you run, look at low-impact aerobics as an alternative. Yoga movements can aggravate your neck if they require bending or twisting your neck. Patients who have problems with the structures in the neck, whether the disc, facet, or nerve, who want to do exercises like yoga should modify or avoid the positions that may involve twisting and turning of the neck. Swimming can irritate the neck because of the turning of the head as you swim. Instead of swimming, I recommend that patients who want to use a pool for exercise walk laps in the pool. If you do want to swim, use a snorkel so that your neck stays in a neutral position.

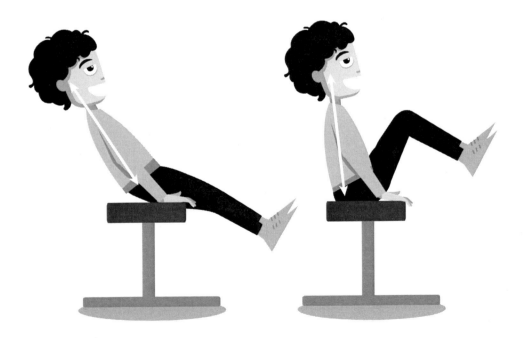

PICTURE 143

Sitting abdominal crunch.

EXERCISES FOR CERVICAL FACET PAIN

Exercises for the neck for patients with cervical facet pain are the same as those described under the cervical disc section *except* that you should not do the neck extension exercise in Picture 133. The extension exercise that involves arching your neck back may aggravate the cervical facets. The best exercises for strengthening the neck if you have had pain due to the inflammation of your cervical facet should be isometric exercises with minimal movement of the spine.

I do not advocate using cervical traction if your pain is coming from your facets. The cervical traction may aggravate the facets, because traction will straighten your neck, which may put more pressure on your facet joints.

Thoracic Spine

THORACIC SPINE BODY POSTURE AND MECHANICS
Thoracic disc or nerve

Most thoracic pain is due either to inflammation inside the thoracic disc or irritation of the thoracic nerve. This type of pain will be aggravated by bending forward, which will either place more pressure on the inside of the disc or create pressure on the outside of the disc, which in turn will irritate the nerve. **Picture 144** will remind you where the thoracic spine is located, primarily in the middle of the back.

The proper posture for patients who have had problems with thoracic disc or nerve pain is to keep that part of your spine in a straight or neutral position, whether you are standing or sitting **(Picture 145)**.

The standing position is much better than the sitting position if you have thoracic disc pain because much less pressure is placed on the disc in the standing position. Make sure you stand up every twenty to thirty minutes whether you are sitting at a desk working or sitting on a sofa watching television. Use a sit-stand desk if you can, because standing is the best position for the thoracic discs (Picture 128). It is essential to bend your knees when you need to reach for something instead of bending over and putting stress on your thoracic discs **(Picture 146)**. If you bend forward at the waist without bending your knees you will increase the pressure on the disc, but if you bend your knees and keep your back straight, no extra pressure is placed on the disc. Practicing good posture will reduce the chance of irritating the inside of the disc or the nerve.

If you cannot bend your knees, then sit down to do the things you need to do such as emptying the washing machine. Use assist devices, such as grabber sticks, which can pick things up off the floor for you if you cannot bend your knees. This also holds true for patients who have osteoporosis or have had compression fractures in their thoracic spine. Keeping the thoracic spine straight will decrease the force on the vertebrae and bones of the spine, consequently decreasing the chances of damaging the bones.

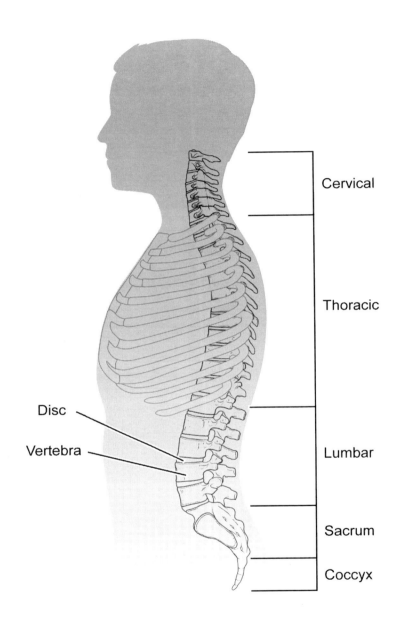

Cervical

Thoracic

Disc

Vertebra

Lumbar

Sacrum

Coccyx

PICTURE 144

Thoracic discs in the front of the spine.

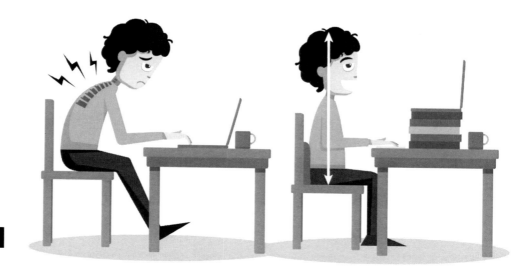

PICTURE 145

No slumping!

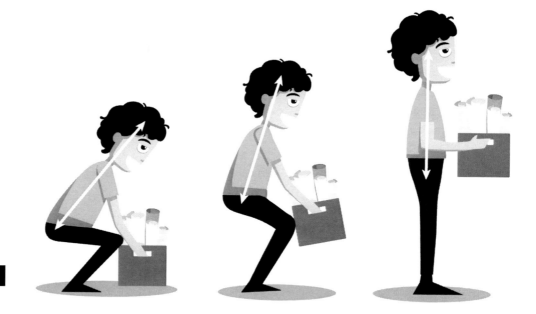

PICTURE 146

Keeping the thoracic
spine straight while
lifting.

Thoracic facets

The patient who has pain originating from the thoracic facet joints will usually hurt with the exact opposite motion as the patient who has pain originating in the discs. Because the facets are in the back of the spine, they will press on each other when you arch or twist your upper back.

The patient with inflamed thoracic facet joints will have a hard time sitting up straight and will feel better in a slumped-over position. This is exactly the opposite of thoracic disc pain patients, who feel better when they are sitting up straight or arching their back. If you have had pain due to inflamed thoracic facets, you will also be more comfortable moving around or sitting than standing in one place. Do not sleep on your back or stomach, which will aggravate your discomfort. You should sleep lying on your side in a fetal position, because that will keep your inflamed facets from pressing on each other. The best way to keep these joints from getting re-aggravated is to avoid the things that involve a lot of twisting or arching of your back.

EXERCISES FOR THORACIC DISC AND NERVE PAIN

An exercise that may decrease your pain from a thoracic disc or nerve problem is an extension exercise that will push the disc away from the nerve. This is the same thing as arching your upper back, which will open up the space for the thoracic discs. Sit on a chair and place your hands on the back of your neck. Then extend your upper back for a couple of seconds before relaxing your posture. You can repeat this as many times as you want. This exercise also will teach you not to slump forward while you are sitting (**Picture 147**).

Exercises for the thoracic spine primarily involve strengthening two major muscle groups, your legs and the core muscles around the thoracic spine, including your abdominal muscles. By getting your legs stronger, you can keep your thoracic spine straight by bending your knees as you do your daily activities. This is best accomplished using a stationary bike because you can increase leg strength with minimal motion of your thoracic spine. You can also use an elliptical trainer or StairMaster to strengthen your legs. Another exercise to build leg strength as well as your core muscles is to walk in a pool with the water up to your mid-chest. As you walk against the water, you will strengthen the muscles in your torso. You also can walk backward through the water, which helps the strengthening process. But no twisting of your back! Walking in water allows very little movement of the thoracic spine, while the thoracic musculature that surrounds the spine is strengthened. You can also use weight machines to strengthen your legs. There are sample leg exercises in the lumbar section that are spine safe.

It is important to strengthen the back muscles, because these muscles will hold you erect without slumping and, in turn, prevent the thoracic disc

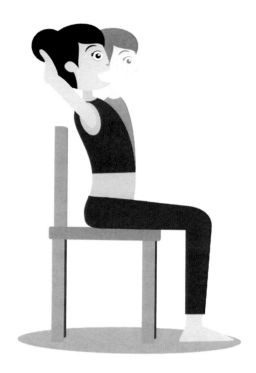

Extension exercise for the thoracic spine.

from becoming inflamed or irritating the nerve. Pull-downs with palms facing away from you and rows are two effective exercises (**Pictures 148** and **149**). Make sure that the back stays completely straight during both of these exercises. If you want to use a rowing machine, make sure that your back stays straight while you are rowing. Do not lean forward!

I recommend that patients limit the twisting or forward bending of their thoracic spine when they exercise. Instead of doing sit-ups to strengthen the abdominal muscles, which may involve bending the thoracic spine, a better exercise is an isometric abdominal muscle contraction (**Picture 150**). You can sit, stand, or lie down to do this exercise. You place your hand over your stomach muscles and then contract your stomach muscles. Hold for five seconds and then relax. Do as many as you want. Once you get used to doing this exercise, you do not need to keep your hands over your stomach muscles.

Another good exercise for your abdominal muscles is the McGill curl-up (**Picture 151**). Lie on your back on the floor with your right leg straight and your left knee bent with your left foot flat on the ground. You then place your hands palm down on the floor underneath the natural curve in your lower back. Contract your abdominal muscles and then slowly raise your head and shoulders off the floor without bending your spine. Hold for a count of five seconds. After doing a few repetitions, repeat this exercise with your right leg bent and your left leg straight.

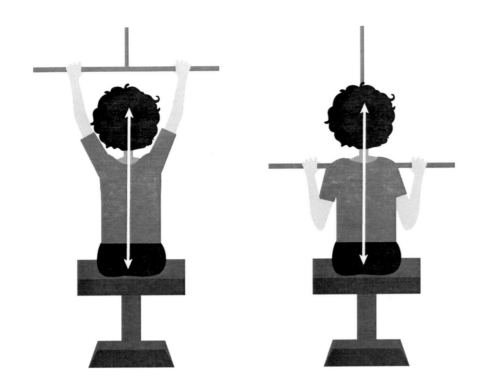

PICTURE 148

Back pull-downs with palms facing away from you.

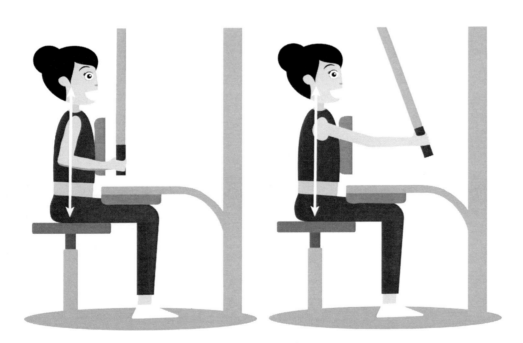

PICTURE 149

Back rows.

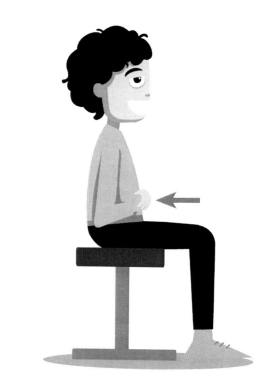

PICTURE 150

Isometric abdominal muscle contraction.

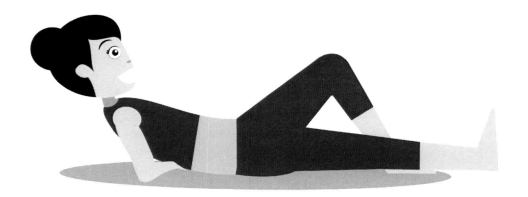

PICTURE 151

The McGill curl-up.

EXERCISES FOR THORACIC FACET PAIN

All the exercises that I mentioned in the section on thoracic discs also are appropriate for patients with thoracic facet problems *except* for the extension exercise (Picture 147), which would aggravate the facets. Be careful with any exercises such as swimming or certain yoga positions that involve arching or twisting of the spine as they could aggravate the thoracic facets.

LUMBAR SPINE

LUMBAR SPINE BODY POSTURE AND MECHANICS

Lumbar disc or nerve

If the lumbar disc or nerve is or was creating your pain, the easiest way to discuss the body mechanics, positions, and exercises is to remember where the disc and nerve sit in the spine. In **Picture 152**, note that the disc and nerve are located in the *front* of the lumbar spine, and the facets or joints are in the *back* of the spine.

Posture and body mechanics can play a large role in preventing recurrences of pain. Because the discs and nerves are located in the front of the spine, they may be aggravated by activities that involve bending forward without bending your knees (**Picture 153**).

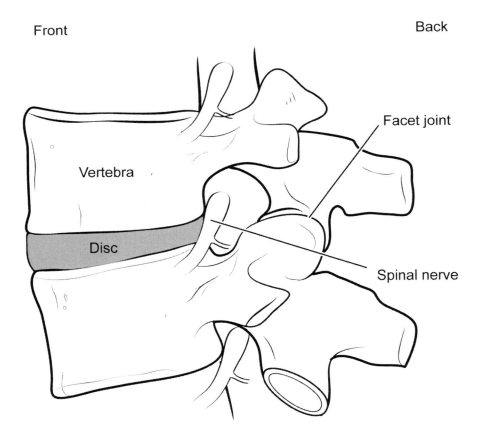

Front

Back

Facet joint

Vertebra

Disc

Spinal nerve

PICTURE 152

Disc and nerve in front of the spine and facet in the back of the spine.

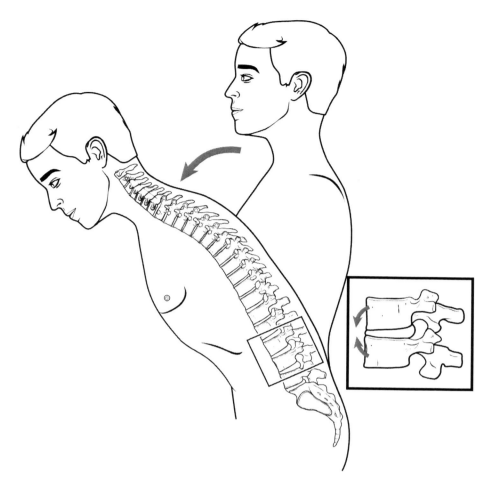

PICTURE 153

Bending forward,
which puts pressure
on the disc.

This incorrect motion will increase the pressure inside the disc, which in turn may at some point inflame the disc and irritate the nerve. So every time you do things such as empty the dishwasher, pick things up off the floor, work in the yard, brush your teeth, or any other of the countless things that you normally do in a bent-forward position, try to find a way to do those activities while keeping your spine straight (**Picture 154**). Sit down or kneel if you have to for a few minutes to do certain chores before bending your back.

The same motion should be used when you are picking things up. Remember, the more you bend the knees and keep the back straight, the less pressure will be applied to the disc and subsequently the nerve.

Twisting activities of the spine can also aggravate the disc, because the rotational movement can create inflammation inside and outside the disc. Always remember to turn your whole body instead of twisting your spine.

The sitting position allows all your body weight and gravity to be placed on top of the disc. This increased pressure can create inflammation inside the disc, or the disc itself may inflame the nerve. Also note the stretching of the nerves in the lumbar spine when your leg is bent in the sitting position compared with when you are standing (**Picture 155**).

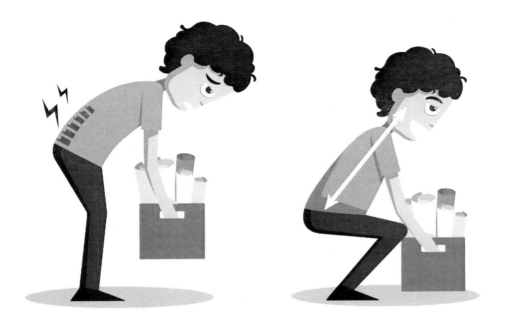

PICTURE 154

Bending with your back versus bending your knees.

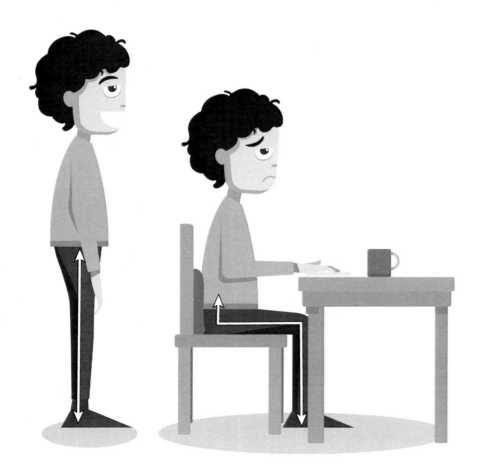

PICTURE 155

Stretching of the nerve in the sitting position.

The sitting position, due to the combination of the increased pressure on the disc and the stretching of the nerve, is the worst position for the spine to be in for long periods of time. This holds true for any part of the spine, whether it is your cervical, thoracic, or lumbar spine.

The basic idea is to keep moving as much as possible. If you do have a job that involves a lot of sitting, ensure that you get up every twenty or thirty minutes and move around so that you don't put prolonged pressure on the disc or irritate the nerve. If you can, use a sit-stand desk that will allow you to work standing up. This will help if you have a history of disc or nerve problems in the lumbar spine. Remember, I am talking about patients with disc and nerve problems who feel more comfortable standing with an erect spine. At times, a disc herniation can create more problems in the center of the spine, resulting in spinal stenosis. The patient with spinal stenosis or facet pain will find the standing position irritating.

If you are driving long distances, ensure that you keep your back up against the seat of the car and do not lean forward. Make sure that you get out of the car and walk around every hour or so. If you are a passenger, put the seat back, because that will keep the full weight of your body off the discs and also will take the tension off the nerve (**Picture 156**).

As you can see in Picture 156, the worst position for your disc and nerve is sitting leaning forward. As you lean back, the pressure in the disc is reduced as is the stretch on the nerve. The standing position puts the least pressure on the disc and the nerve.

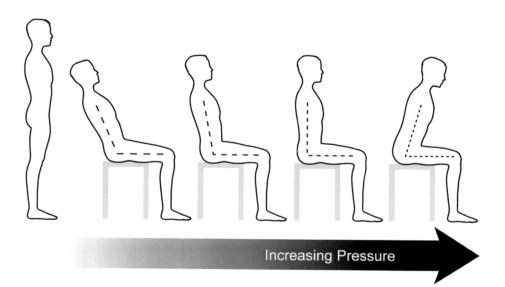

PICTURE 156

Driver and passenger positions.

Increasing Pressure

Lumbar facets

The lumbar facets, as you can see in **Picture 157**, are located in the *back* of the spine, in contrast to the disc and nerve in the front of the spine.

Picture 157 illustrates that as you bend forward the facets separate, and when you bend backward (extension), the joints press on each other. The motion of bending backward can create pain if your facet joints are inflamed. When you stand in one place or lie flat on your back, your lumbar

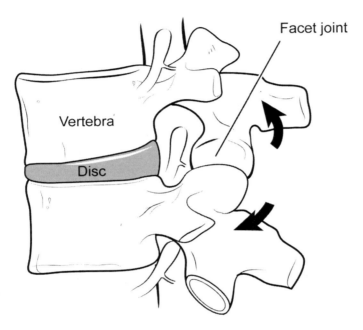

Flexion (bending forward)

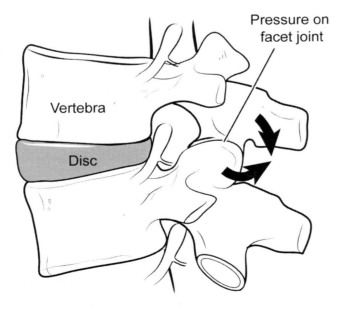

Extension
(arching the back or bending backward)

PICTURE 157

Facet joints open when you bend forward and press on each other when you bend backward.

spine goes into an extension position because of the natural arched curve in the lumbar spine. This is why standing in one place and lying on your back can create increased pain if your facets are inflamed. You may notice that your pain from the facets will be better once you start to walk and lean forward, and/or if you sleep curled up on your side in a fetal position, because the facet joints open up in these positions.

If you have had a problem with facet pain, try to use your legs to bend, instead of using your back. Because the facets are located in the back of the spine, they may open up as you bend forward, but as you straighten back up, the joints can come in contact with each other. So every time you do things such as picking up a child, getting dressed, doing your hair, or putting on makeup, bend your knees or kneel so that your back stays fairly straight. If you cannot do either, sit down to do these daily activities.

Because you do not want to arch your back, which is the same thing as putting your back into an extension position, you should not sit with a lumbar support if you have been diagnosed with a facet problem. The lumbar support will create an arch in your back. So deflate the car lumbar support and do not use an office chair with one of those supports. Sitting for long periods of time may not create a problem as it would with patients with disc pain, unless you sit completely erect, which may irritate the joints. Patients with a history of facet problems do better when they sit slumped over a little bit.

Standing in one position will create pressure on your facets, so if you are on your feet a lot, make sure that you continue to move around instead of standing in one place. If you use a sit-stand desk and have had recent problems with your facets, you should sit more than stand because that will keep the pressure off the joints. Minimize twisting motions of your back as they can aggravate your joints. Move your whole body instead of rotating your back.

An important difference between the joints and the discs is the position in which you sleep. If you have a problem with your facets, you do not want to have your back completely straight when you sleep, because that position will create pressure on your facet joints. You should sleep on your side, curled up in a fetal position. This will keep your joints open, compared with sleeping on your back or stomach, which can aggravate your joints because of the extension position of your spine. Patients ask me about buying certain types of mattresses that may be better than others. I am not sure there really is much difference, but if you are going to spend your money on sleep aids, I would recommend an electric hospital-type bed frame (**Picture 158**). In this type of bed, you can raise the back up, so that you can sleep on your back without having your spine in an extension position. This slightly upright position will keep your facets open and will allow you to sleep on your back.

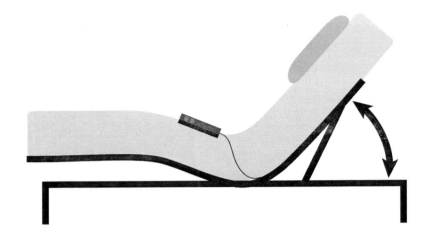

PICTURE 158

Electric bed that allows you to raise the back up to take pressure off the facet joints.

EXERCISES FOR LUMBAR DISC AND NERVE PAIN

Most exercises for lumbar disc and nerve pain should consist primarily of strengthening the stomach, leg, and back muscles without moving the spine. A back extension is the one exercise in which movement of the spine will help relieve the pressure of the disc and the nerve **(Picture 159)**. This motion will open up the space where the disc is located and therefore also move the disc away from the nerve.

I usually tell patients to do back extensions several times a day as part of their daily exercise regimen, even during the time that they are hurting. This is a good exercise to do during the time you have pain coming from the disc

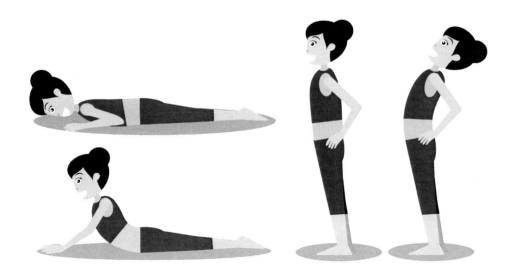

PICTURE 159

Back extensions done lying down and standing.

or the nerve, because it may decrease some of your discomfort. It works the same way a lumbar support in your car does by giving the disc more space.

The machine back extension replicates the back extension but you can build more muscle because of being able to use weight (**Picture 160**). Notice that there is no bending forward.

I also suggest pull-down exercises as shown in **Picture 161** to build your back muscles. Keep your palms facing toward you, because that will make you arch your back and open up your disc spaces.

Another good exercise for your lower back is the back row as seen in **Picture 162**. Keep your back straight as you row so that you do not compress your discs.

I recommend using weight machines to strengthen your legs, but if you have had lumbar disc and nerve problems, stay away from the leg press, squats with weights, and full leg extensions, because all of these involve either creating pressure on the disc or pulling on the nerve. Here are some sample leg exercises to do that are spine safe.

Leg curls can be done lying on a bench with your back straight (**Picture 163**).

The standing calf raise is a good exercise if you have had disc and nerve pain. It allows your disc space to open as you rise up on your toes, because you will tend to arch your back as you rise up (**Picture 164**). And it strengthens your legs at the same time. Once your leg pain is gone, you can hold some dumbbells while you are doing this exercise.

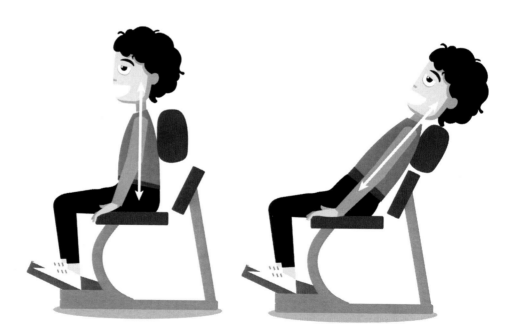

PICTURE 160

Machine back extension.

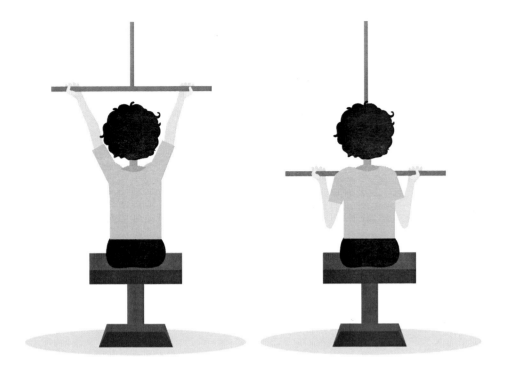

PICTURE 161

Back pull-downs with palms facing you.

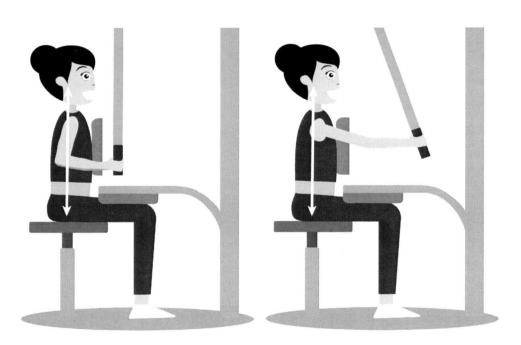

PICTURE 162

Back rows.

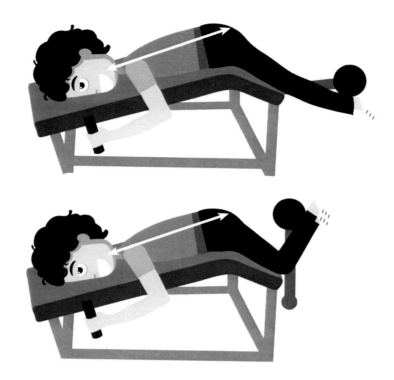

PICTURE 163

Leg curls.

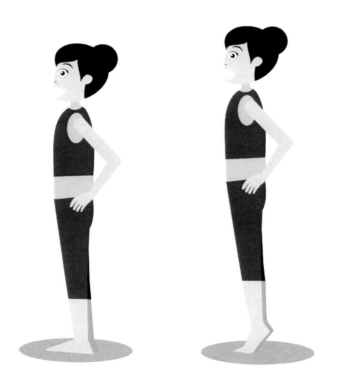

PICTURE 164

Standing calf raises.

Wall squats against a wall are a good exercise to build your leg muscles, but make sure you stop before you get to ninety degrees (**Picture 165**). They are called wall squats because instead of placing weight on your shoulders, you just have some air on your shoulders. You want to stop before you get to what would be the sitting position. This will minimize the stretch on the nerve. I usually recommend doing this exercise if you are having only back pain, with no leg pain.

Leg extensions are an exercise that I am asked about all the time. It is not my favorite exercise for leg strengthening, because if you straighten the legs completely, you may pull on your lumbar nerve roots, which is *not* good if you have had leg pain recently. If you really want to do this exercise, wait until your buttock or leg pain is completely gone. When you do this exercise, stop at forty-five degrees, which is about half-way to a full extension of your legs (**Picture 166**).

The exercises for the patient with lumbar disc or nerve pain should involve strengthening the stomach and back muscles without bending or twisting the lumbar spine. The following are several exercises for the abdominal muscles which do not involve bending the back. The first one is an isometric abdominal muscle contraction (**Picture 167**). You can sit, stand, or lie down to do this exercise. You place your hand over your stomach muscles and then contract your stomach muscles. Hold for five seconds and then relax. You can do as many as you want, whether driving in a car or standing in one place.

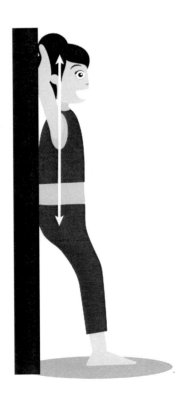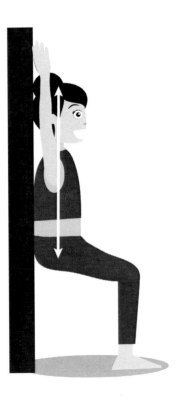

PICTURE 165

Wall squats against a wall, stopping before you get to ninety degrees.

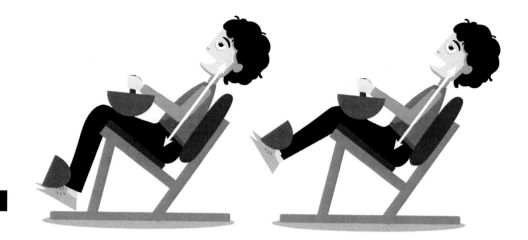

PICTURE 166

Leg extension stopping at forty-five degrees.

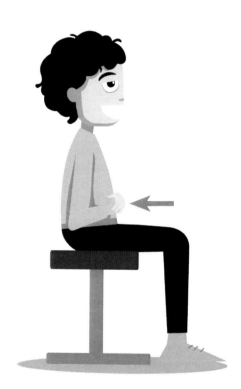

PICTURE 167

Isometric abdominal muscle contraction.

The next abdominal exercise is a McGill curl-up **(Picture 168)**. Lie on your back on the floor with your right leg straight and your left knee bent with your left foot flat on the ground. You then place your hands palm down on the floor underneath the natural curve in your lower back. Contract your abdominal muscles and then slowly raise your head and shoulders off the floor without bending your spine. Hold for a count of five seconds. After doing a few repetitions, you can then repeat this exercise with your right leg bent and your left leg straight.

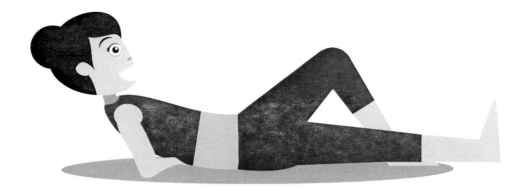

The McGill curl-up.

Plank holds are also a good exercise to do if you have a problem with your disc and nerve because your spine stays straight **(Picture 169)**. Once you get in the position seen in the picture, you can contract your abdominal muscles for twenty seconds and then relax for a minute before repeating the contraction. You can do sets of ten and then, as your abdominals become stronger, you can contract your abdominal muscles for a longer period of time.

Notice that I did not mention sit-ups or the use of abdominal machines. Both of these exercises make you bend your lumbar spine forward, which increases the pressure in the discs.

Traction and the use of an inversion table for the patient with lumbar disc and nerve pain can be helpful at times. Yoga is probably not a suitable exercise for patients with lumbar degenerative disc disease because of

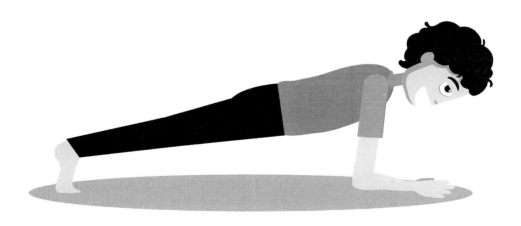

PICTURE 169

Plank holds.

the twisting and bending of the spine. If you simply do not want to give up yoga, avoid positions that involve bending forward and twisting the lower spine. The cobra pose in yoga is actually a great back-strengthening exercise, which also pushes the disc away from the nerve.

The best aerobic exercise for the patient with a lumbar disc or nerve problem is walking. This will help build your legs so that you use them instead of your back in your daily activities. Even better would be to walk in a pool in waist-deep water. The advantage of walking in water is that it provides more of an isometric exercise for your stomach and lower back muscles than walking on land, and at the same time it unloads the weight off the discs. Walking forward and then backward in the pool is usually the first step in strengthening the legs, back, and stomach muscles. This can be done even if you are having pain because walking actually takes the pressure off your discs.

Swimming is good for patients with disc or nerve problems as long as you avoid flip turns at the end of the pool. You can also use a treadmill or any other nonimpact aerobic equipment, such as an elliptical trainer or StairMaster. Try to use these machines without bending forward.

Riding a bike, whether outdoors or stationary, is also a good exercise, as long as you do not have any significant residual sciatic nerve pain. If you use a stationary bike, you may be better off with a recumbent bike instead of an upright bike, particularly if your previous leg pain was worse in the sitting position, as the recumbent bike will let you slide forward in the bike seat, which will take some pressure off the disc as well as reduce tension on the nerve (**Picture 170**).

If you do use an outdoor bike, use a bike that keeps you upright, so that you are not bent over from the waist.

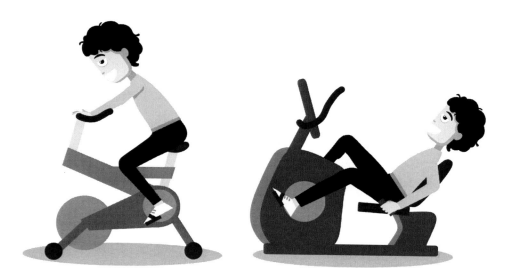

PICTURE 170

Upright bike versus recumbent bike.

I am not a big fan of running, because it creates a certain amount of pounding of the disc. We now are starting to see that walking provides health benefits as good as if not better than running offers. But if you are one of those people who cannot stop running, my advice is to wait at least several weeks after your back or leg pain is gone, and then walk for a couple of weeks before returning to running.

EXERCISES FOR LUMBAR FACET PAIN

If your problem is with your lumbar facets, the exercises I recommend consist of strengthening the stomach, leg, and back muscles without moving the spine. One exercise that may relieve your facet pain is a rotating of your pelvis so that your buttocks are tucked under your spine (**Picture 171**).

This exercise will take the arch out of your spine and give your facets more room. I do this exercise all the time because I am slightly swaybacked, and therefore I am prone to pain from my facets. You should not do an extension exercise such as seen in Picture 159. This exercise will create more pressure on your facet joints.

Another good exercise to do is pull-downs, which will strengthen your upper back muscles. Make sure that you position your hands so that your palms are facing away from you as that will keep you from arching your back as you pull down (**Picture 172**).

You also can do rows using a pulley system, as seen in **Picture 173**, but ensure that you lean forward slightly so that no pressure is placed on your lumbar facets.

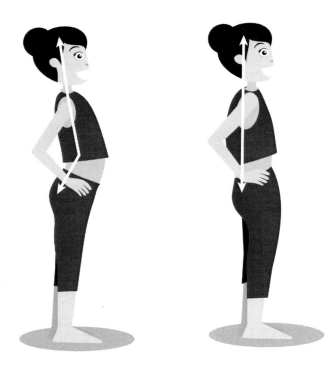

PICTURE 171

Rotation of pelvis so that your buttocks are tucked under your spine.

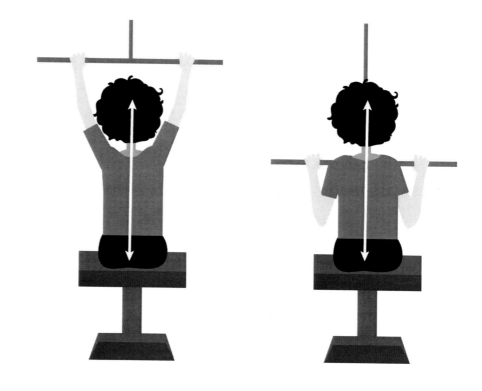

Back pull-downs with palms facing away from you.

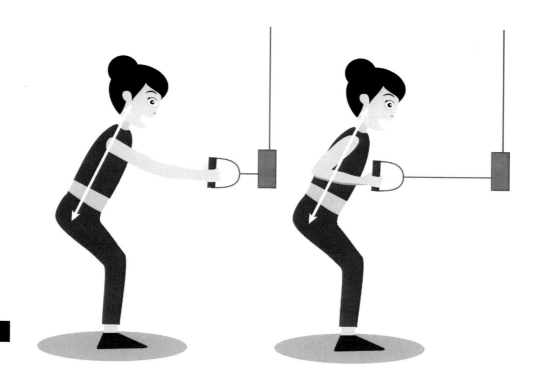

Back rows while bending forward slightly.

You can also do rows sitting, but do not let your back arch or straighten up as you do this exercise.

For your legs, you can do the two exercises that I showed you for disc problems, the leg curls in Picture 163 and the leg extension in Picture 166. Do *not* do the standing calf raises shown in Picture 164 or the wall squats shown in Picture 165, because both create an arch in your back that may aggravate your facets. Instead of doing standing calf raises, you can do calf raises in a sitting position (**Picture 174**). You can put dumbbells on your knees as you do your calf raises.

To strengthen your abdominal muscles, you can do isometric abdominal muscle contractions as shown in **Picture 175**. You can sit, stand, or lie down to do this exercise. You place your hand over your stomach muscles and then contract your stomach muscles. Hold for five seconds and then relax.

Another favorite abdominal exercise that I would recommend is the sitting abdominal crunch (**Picture 176**). While sitting on a bench, contract your stomach muscles first and then slowly bring your knees up. Hold for a couple of seconds and then bring your knees down but do not let your feet touch the floor. Repeat this repetition ten times to start with and then rest.

Do not do the plank holds for the abdomen as shown in Picture 169 because the straight spine position can aggravate your facet pain. The inversion table will make your pain worse if your back pain is due to inflamed facets, because the inversion table creates a straightening of the spine. You can do most aerobic exercises, but avoid running as that may aggravate the facet joints. You should not walk on a treadmill in an inclined position, because

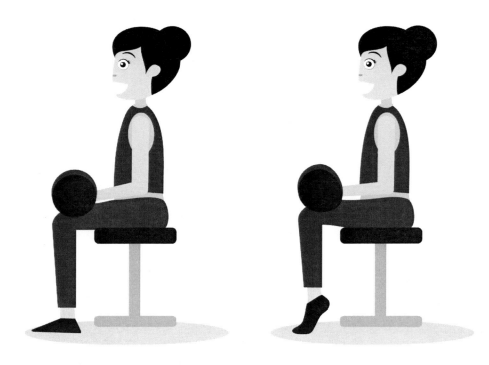

PICTURE 174

Sitting calf raises.

that will create an arch in your spine and may aggravate your facet joint. Walking, biking, and using an elliptical machine are all good ways to exercise without irritating your facet joints. The position of the spine while you are swimming is usually one of arching the back, which can aggravate the spine if there is a problem with your facets or joints. Therefore, it would be better to walk in the pool instead of swim.

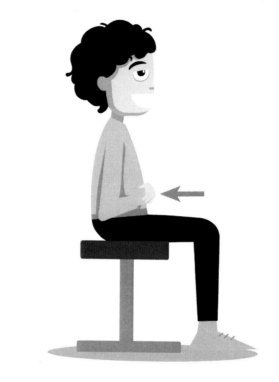

PICTURE 175

Isometric abdominal muscle contractions.

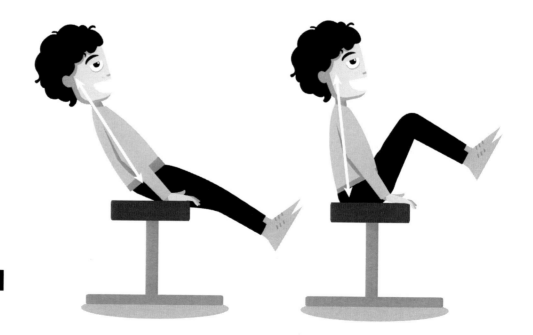

PICTURE 176

Sitting abdominal crunch.

LUMBAR SPINAL STENOSIS

LUMBAR SPINAL STENOSIS BODY POSTURE AND MECHANICS

The posture and body mechanics for lumbar spinal stenosis are somewhat different from those for other issues in the spine that create back and leg pain. Lumbar spinal stenosis, which was discussed earlier in the book, involves a narrowing of the spinal canal (**Picture 177**). This narrowing usually is due to a combination of the enlargement of the facet joints, thickening of ligaments in the back of the spine, and/or disc herniations.

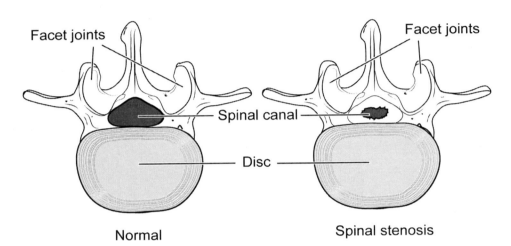

Normal   Spinal stenosis

PICTURE 177

Spinal stenosis.

This narrowing also can occur because of a slippage in the spine called spondylolisthesis, which is shown in **Picture 178**. Spondylolisthesis exists when one of the vertebra slips over the next level, which can create spinal stenosis.

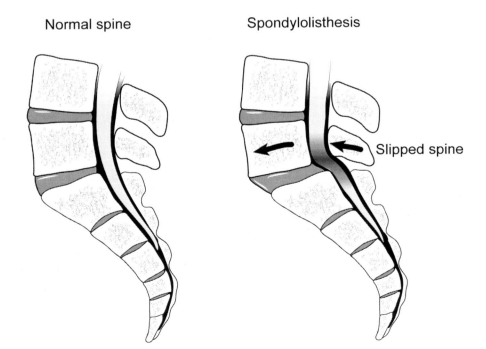

Normal spine   Spondylolisthesis

PICTURE 178

Spinal stenosis caused by spondylolisthesis.

The problem with spinal stenosis starts when the patient with stenosis stands or walks. When all humans stand up straight, the spinal canal narrows because of the natural arch of the spine, no matter whether you have a normal-size spinal canal or the canal is narrowed because of spinal stenosis. This is just a normal physiologic process that happens with all humans. In spinal stenosis, you have a higher chance of irritating the lumbar nerves when you stand up because there is not enough room inside the canal for the nerves **(Picture 179)**.

Walking and standing for long periods of time are not good positions for spinal stenosis patients. You will feel better when you are standing or walking in a bent-forward position as that will open up your spine. If you are going to be on your feet for a while, I recommend that you make it a point to sit down every thirty minutes or so, which may keep your spinal nerves from becoming inflamed.

Spinal stenosis and lumbar facet pain are similar in that both can be aggravated by having your lumbar spine in the extension position. You should not use the lumbar support in your car, which is going to put your back in extension, or sleep on your back or stomach, which will narrow the spinal canal. If you have spinal stenosis, you should sleep on your side, curled up in a fetal position, which will keep your canal open. I even tell patients to stuff a pillow behind their backs while in the fetal position, so that they cannot roll over onto their backs. Otherwise, they will awaken and hurt, and they will have a hard time getting out of bed. If you have a hard time sleeping on your side, you can use a hospital-type electric bed. By raising the back

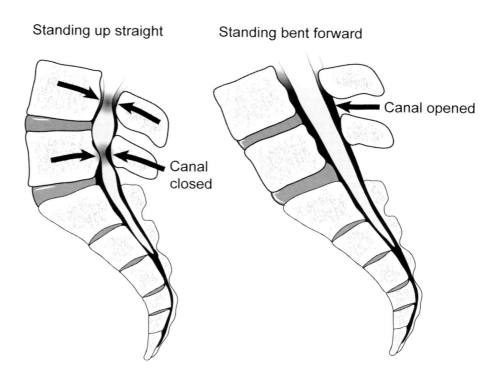

Standing up straight   Standing bent forward

Canal opened

Canal closed

PICTURE 179

Standing up straight creates narrowing of the spinal canal in the spinal stenosis patient.

of the bed, you can sleep in a semi-upright position and therefore keep the spine open, just like sleeping in a recliner. This will allow you to sleep on your back and not awaken with pain.

EXERCISES FOR LUMBAR SPINAL STENOSIS

Aerobic exercise for spinal stenosis patients should involve riding a bicycle or stationary bike, which will not aggravate the spinal stenosis as you are sitting while you are on the bike. I do not recommend walking for exercise or using any form of exercise equipment that involves standing, such as a StairMaster or treadmill, because the upright position may irritate your spinal stenosis. If you really enjoy one of these forms of exercises, stop after twenty minutes and sit down for five minutes. Save your walking for fun. When you do walk, sit down for five minutes once every thirty minutes that you walk. This will keep the nerves in your spine from becoming aggravated. Swimming also is not a good form of exercise, because the swimming position puts the spinal stenosis patient into an extension position, which will narrow your canal and possibly irritate the nerves. You can walk in the pool against the water, but stop every thirty minutes and sit down for several minutes to eliminate the possibility of irritating the nerves. The inversion table will make your pain worse if your back pain is due to spinal stenosis, because the inversion table creates a straightening of the spine.

There are a few exercises for spinal stenosis that may make you feel better while you are in pain. These flexion exercises which round your back will open your spinal canal and give your nerves room to breathe. One example is the back flexion exercise shown in **Picture 180**. Start by lying on the floor and pulling your knees to your chest. Keep pulling your knees until you feel a light stretch. Hold for five to ten seconds and put your feet back on the floor. Repeat after a few minutes. This back flexion exercise can also be done by sitting in a chair and just bending forward from the waist. Hold for five to ten seconds and then straighten up. Repeat after a few minutes.

Another exercise that will help open your spinal canal is the pelvic tilt **(Picture 181)**. Lie on your back and keep your knees bent up. Squeeze your stomach as if you are trying to push your bellybutton down toward the floor. This will push your lower back down toward the floor as your pelvis tilts forward. Do not push down with your legs as that may cause you to arch your back.

If you have spinal stenosis, I would recommend that you do exercises to strengthen your back, abdomen, and legs, but they have to be done in a way that does not aggravate your underlying condition. You should do most exercises in a sitting position, and do not do any exercises that involve arching or bending backward. For instance, avoid exercises like back extensions and plank holds.

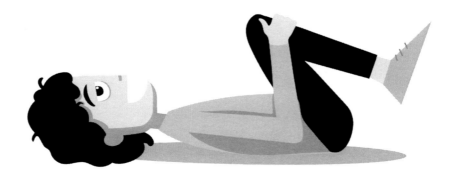

PICTURE 180

Knees to chest
flexion.

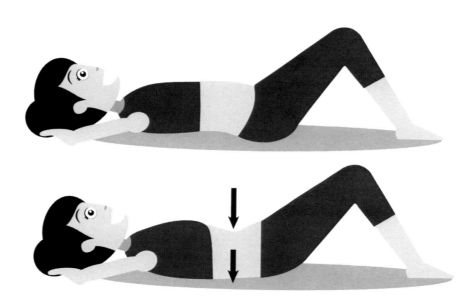

PICTURE 181

Pelvic tilts.

A good back exercise to do is pull-downs, which will strengthen your upper back muscles. Stand up to grab the bar and then sit down. Make sure that you position your hands so that your palms are facing away from you, as that will keep you from arching your back as you pull down **(Picture 182)**. As you pull down, let your back roll into a ball, thus opening up your spinal canal.

Another good exercise for your lower back is the back rows as seen in **Picture 183**.

To strengthen your abdominal muscles, you can do isometric abdominal muscle contractions as shown in **Picture 184**. Place your hand over your stomach muscles and then contract your stomach muscles. Hold for five seconds and then relax. You can do this exercise while sitting or lying down; stenosis patients should refrain from doing this exercise while standing.

Another favorite abdominal exercise that I recommend is the sitting abdominal crunch (**Picture 185**). While sitting on a bench, contract your stomach muscles first and then slowly bring your knees up. Hold for a couple

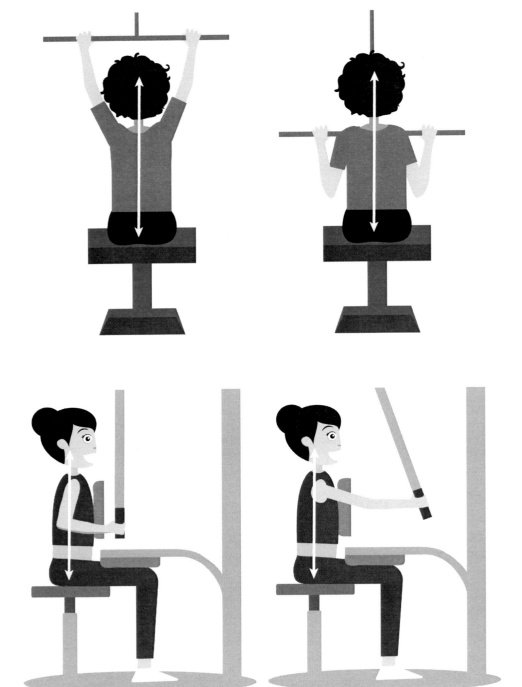

PICTURE 182

Back pull-downs with palms facing away from you.

PICTURE 183

Back rows.

of seconds and then bring your knees down but do not let your feet touch the floor. Repeat this repetition ten times to start with and then rest.

The best exercise to strengthen your legs is a stationary bike, whether it is an upright or a recumbent bike (**Picture 186**). Either bike will work, so pick the one you feel most comfortable on.

You can also use exercise machines to strengthen your legs. Leg curls can be done lying on a bench (**Picture 187**).

Sitting calf raises will also strengthen your legs without aggravating your spinal stenosis (**Picture 188**). You can put dumbbells on your knees as you do your calf raises.

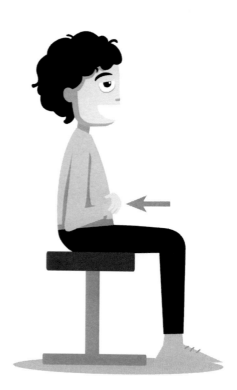

PICTURE 184

Isometric abdominal muscle contractions.

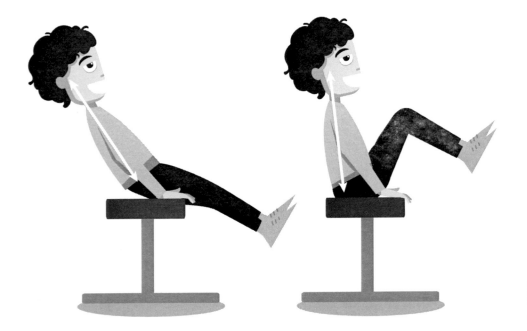

PICTURE 185

Sitting abdominal crunch.

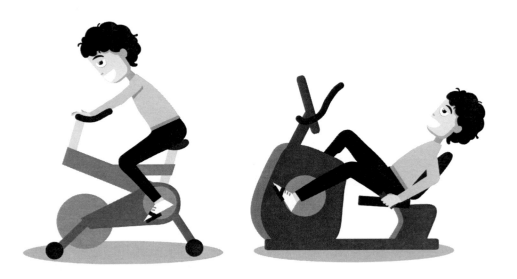

PICTURE 186

Upright bike versus recumbent bike.

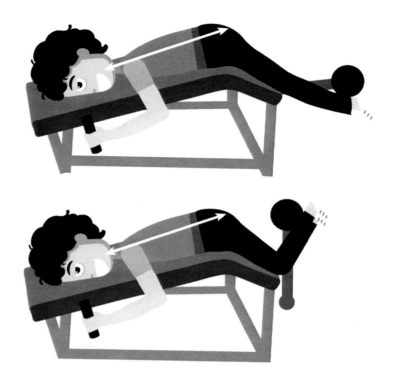

PICTURE 187

Leg curls.

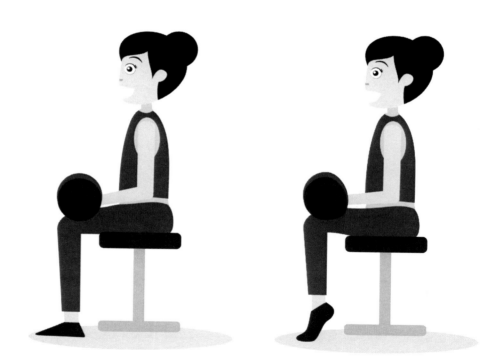

PICTURE 188

Sitting calf raises.

Leg extension exercises usually do not aggravate spinal stenosis if you limit the extension to forty-five degrees, which is about half-way to a full extension of your legs (**Picture 189**). Do not straighten your legs completely to ninety degrees. Do this exercise when you do not have any leg pain.

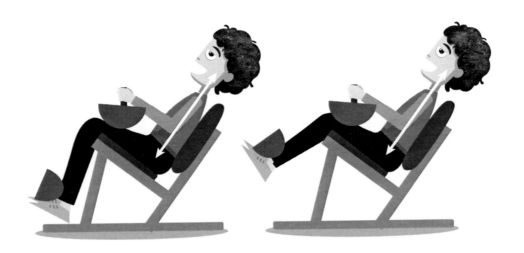

PICTURE 189

Leg extension stopping at forty-five degrees.

SUMMARY

1. The **Straight Spine Safe Spine** Program gives you exercises that may decrease your pain.

2. The **Straight Spine Safe Spine** Program teaches you body positions and mechanics that will keep you from aggravating your spine.

3. The **Straight Spine Safe Spine** Program shows you how to exercise without inflaming the part of the spine that you are having problems with.

4. The **Straight Spine Safe Spine** Program is designed for each *specific* problem that may be creating your pain.

5. The **Straight Spine Safe Spine** Program is the start to a long-term lifestyle change to prevent recurrences of pain.

I end this chapter with one last picture that I want you to always remember (**Picture 190**). The more you keep your spine straight, the less you will need to read this book.

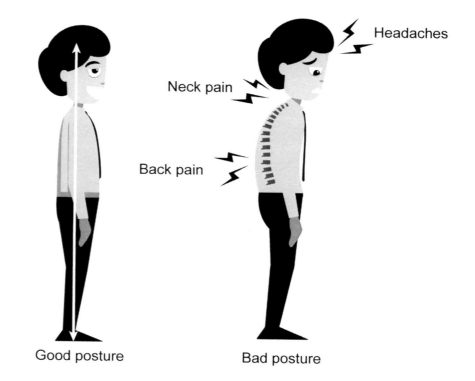

Headaches

Neck pain

Back pain

Good posture   Bad posture

PICTURE 190

Straight spine,
less pain.

> **Remember: Straight Spine Safe Spine.**

Still have questions? The last chapter offers answers to questions I am most often asked by patients.

CHAPTER 18

Answers to the Most Common Questions Patients Ask Me

Patients have often asked me the same questions through the years while they have dealt with their spine pain. These are the most common questions that I am asked in no certain order.

Remember this is my view on these subjects, and it is only one view!

1. Does laser surgery for the spine really exist?

I happen to work in one of the largest medical centers in the world with a group of extremely talented orthopedic spine and neurosurgeons, who all are well trained in the latest techniques, and not a single one of them uses a laser to operate on the spine. *Why don't they perform laser spine surgery?* They would if a laser could be safely used to operate on the spine and be beneficial to the patient at the same time. But because of technical and safety issues, the laser is not usually used for spine surgery. If you look really closely at all the websites and television ads, you will find that this is mostly a marketing ploy. The facilities advertise laser surgery, but then actually perform the same surgeries that most competent spine surgeons and neurosurgeons do. Before you use these facilities, I recommend that you get something in writing from them that states exactly how the laser is going to be used for your care.

I should also mention that some of these facilities use a procedure called radiofrequency thermocoagulation (RFTC) and sometimes refer to it as laser surgery. It is not laser surgery and it is not used for spine surgery. It is primarily a pain management procedure that is used to mask the pain. I will talk about RFTC in the next question. Also, beware of the laser places that do multiple procedures on several successive days. They may start with facet blocks, epidurals, nerve root blocks, and/or RFTC and end with back surgery. It takes several weeks for any of these procedures to have their full effect. You are better off waiting several weeks between procedures to see if you get relief before moving on to the next procedure.

2. Would a procedure called radiofrequency thermocoagulation (RFTC), which involves burning nerves, work for me?

This procedure is designed to be used only for patients with facet pain who do not obtain long-term relief from facet blocks. The nerves that go to the facet joints can be heated or so-called "burned" so that you do not feel the pain from inflamed facet joints. I have done this procedure for many years, but rarely have to use it because most patients respond to just placing steroids *inside* the inflamed facet joint. I do this procedure on patients only as a last resort, because RFTC merely masks the pain by burning the nerves. If you cannot feel the pain and continue to use bad body mechanics, you are going to risk creating degeneration of the facet joint. It makes a lot more sense to eliminate the inflammation inside the facet joint and then learn proper body mechanics, so that you do not re-inflame the joint.

Another problem is that RFTC is used at times for patients who do *not* have facet pain. Facet pain in the back and neck *never* goes down the arm or leg. The only structure in the spine that can create pain going down the arm or leg is an inflamed nerve from your spine. These are the nerves that also give you the ability to use your arms and legs. These are *not* the nerves to the facet joints. You *cannot* burn these nerves. The only procedures you can have done on these inflamed nerves is a nerve root block or epidural. What happens frequently is that patients will have nerve pain going down the arm or leg and will have a facet block. Even though the arm or leg pain does not go away, these patients will then have an RFTC of the facet joints. And still have pain after the procedure. You have to treat the right structure in the right way to get pain relief. I address the issue of doing the right procedure for the right problem in question five.

I mentioned earlier that the best way to treat the facet joints is by placing the steroids *inside* the facet joint. To properly eliminate inflammation, you have to put the steroids directly in the area of the inflammation. It often appears that physicians who do facet blocks put the steroids on the *outside* of the facet joints and therefore never eliminate the inflammation. Why? Because it takes training and time to get the steroids *inside* the facet joint. And when you don't get relief from the procedure, the physician will talk about "burning the nerves." I treat thousands of patients every year and do an RFTC for facet joint pain less than a half dozen times a year. Be careful of "burning" nerves. And always ask for the X-ray pictures of your facet blocks, so that the physicians can prove that they actually placed the steroids *inside* the facet joint.

3. Is a muscle or a joint creating my buttock pain?

Pain in the buttock area is one of the most common reasons why patients come to see me, and a lot of them have had different forms of therapy with minimal relief. Buttock pain can be caused by an inflammation of the hip, sacroiliac joint, piriformis muscle, or hamstring muscle, but *most* often buttock pain is due to inflammation of one of the nerves in the lumbar or sacral spine. For example, **Picture 191** shows the areas of the body that will be painful when the L5 nerve is inflamed.

As you can see in Picture 191, the inflamed L5 nerve can cause all structures in the buttock area to be painful, whether it is the sacroiliac joint, the piriformis muscle, or even some of the hamstring muscles. Not because there is anything wrong with the muscle or the joint, but because the inflamed L5 nerve is creating the muscle spasm and pain in the area of the joint. You have to treat the L5 nerve to make your buttock pain go away, not the muscle or

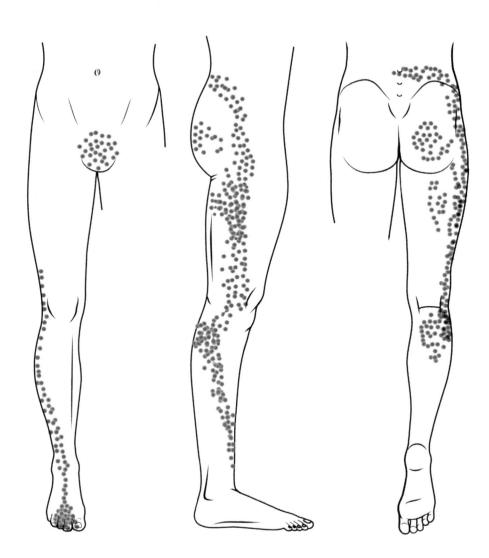

PICTURE 191

Buttock pain because of an inflamed L5 nerve.

the joint in the buttock! If you have buttock pain and therapy is not getting you better, start thinking about the possibility that your buttock pain may be due to a nerve in your lumbar spine.

One more important point. As Picture 191 shows, the L5 nerve starts in the back and then goes to your groin, buttock, hip, and then down your leg. So if the nerve is inflamed due to a disc herniation or a narrowing in your spine, you can have pain in any of these areas. But the pain may not be in all places at the same time. What that means is that you can have buttock pain from the L5 nerve *without* having any leg pain or back pain. One of the most common reasons why medical practitioners start thinking about other diagnoses for buttock pain is that they expect the lumbar nerves to *always* create back and leg pain at the same time the patient is having buttock pain. *Not true!* If you treat the lumbar nerve, the buttock pain will go away. Chapter 12 gives you more information regarding buttock pain.

4. Is bursitis causing the side of my hip to hurt?

There is a bursa, which is a sac of fluid that decreases the friction between tissues, over this part of the hip. This bursa can become inflamed and therefore create pain (**Picture 192**), but it is not usually the reason why the side of your hip hurts.

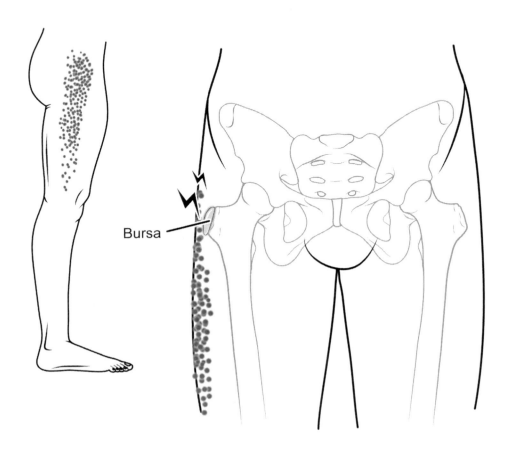

Bursa

Bursa on the side of the hip.

The area around the side of the hip is usually painful because one of the nerves in the lumbar spine is inflamed as a result of a disc herniation or a narrowing of the spinal canal, which in turn inflames the nerve. **Picture 193** shows that the L3, L4, and L5 nerves cover the side of the hip. When the nerves in the lumbar spine are inflamed, they can create pain over the bursa on the side of your hip. Chapter 7 gives you more information regarding hip pain.

5. Why didn't my pain injection work? Are all injections of the spine the same?

I discuss this issue with patients all day long! Not all injections of the spine are the same, and the main reason why you would not get relief from an injection is that the anti-inflammatory steroid medication never gets to the area that is inflamed. The physician *has* to get the medication to the specific

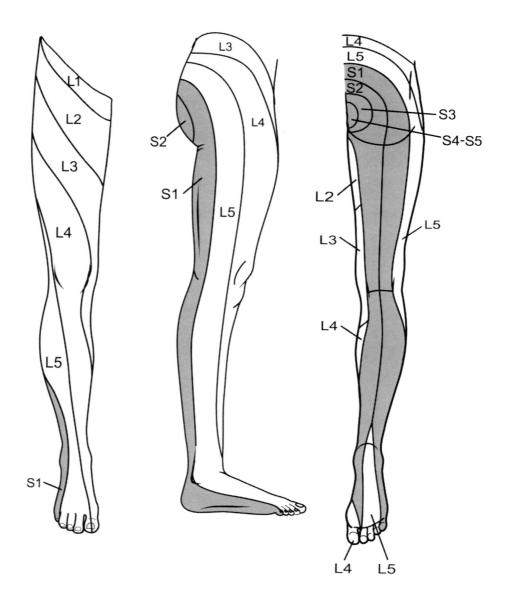

PICTURE 193

Pain in the side of the hip is usually due to inflammation of the lumbar nerves.

structure that is inflamed for it to be beneficial. **Picture 194**, a cross-section of the spine, shows the different areas that create pain on the left-hand side and the specific procedure that needs to be done to treat the problem on the right-hand side.

There are specific procedures for each inflamed structure of the spine:

1. If you have an inflamed annular tear *inside* the disc, your best procedure is an intradiscal steroid injection.

2. If you have an inflamed nerve root due to the irritation of the *outside* of the herniated disc, your best procedure is a nerve root block.

3. If you have an inflamed facet joint, your best procedure is a facet block.

Now what happens if you have an inflamed tear inside your disc and your physician performs an epidural? *Absolutely nothing.* Or what happens if the physician performs a facet block even though your pain is coming from the disc herniation inflaming the nerve root? *Absolutely nothing.* What happens if you are having pain going down your arm or leg because of a disc herniation inflaming the nerve and the physician does an RFTC procedure and burns the nerve to the facets? *Absolutely nothing.*

You have to treat the structure that is inflamed to get pain relief!

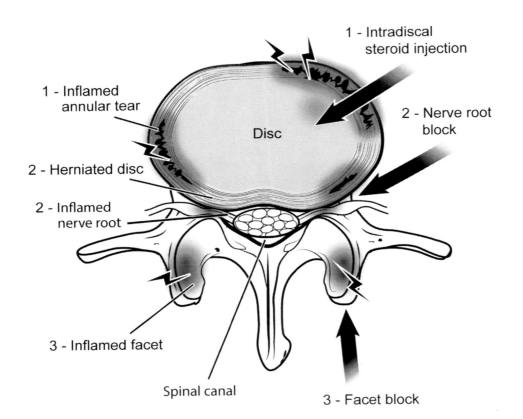

PICTURE 194

Specific procedures for specific areas that create pain.

Because you have to locate the specific structure that is creating your pain, these procedures, whether a nerve root block, facet block, or intradiscal steroid injection, cannot be done without the use of a continuous X-ray machine, also called fluoroscopy, as the practitioner has to be able to see the actual structure that is being treated. I always tell patients to ask for the pictures that are taken by the fluoroscopy machine when they have their procedures. If the physician does not save the pictures from the procedure, it is time to find someone who does. I have made it a point to include the pictures as part of my report for the last twenty years so that I can show the patient exactly what I have done, and I can also pass these pictures along to the surgeon in case the patient needs an operation.

The primary reason the right injections for spine pain are not done for the right problem is due to the lack of training of physicians. You need to make sure that the doctor doing your procedure has been properly trained to do minimally invasive procedures. Most anesthesiology, physical medicine, surgery, or neurology programs do not provide enough training in these procedures, and therefore physicians need to undergo additional training for six months to a year *after* their residency to learn how to do these procedures. Weekend courses do not count. A physician can use weekend courses to refine existing skills, but such courses should not be used to learn these procedures.

6. Is there a chance that my diagnosis of fibromyalgia, neuropathy, and/or restless leg syndrome may actually be due to a problem in my spine?

These conditions present a lot of the same symptoms that you would find in someone who has an inflamed disc, facet joint, or nerve in the spine. Patients with the diagnosis of fibromyalgia, as well as a patient with a herniated disc in the back or neck, may experience pain and muscle spasm in their back, neck, joints, and extremities. The same goes for patients with the diagnosis of neuropathy. These patients may have numbness and burning pain in their legs and feet, which is exactly the same type of pain suffered by patients with sciatic nerve pain because of a problem in the spine. Inflammation of the lumbar nerves due to either spinal stenosis or a disc herniation can create discomfort in the legs and make them "restless" at night. I have seen many patients who have been labeled with one of these three diagnoses who actually had a problem in their spine. The irritation of discs, nerves, and joints can create the exact same symptoms as in fibromyalgia, neuropathies, and restless leg syndrome. You do not want to miss a treatable cause of your pain and have to live with chronic pain!

7. Even though my neck does not hurt, could the pain in my shoulder be coming from my spine?

One of the most common reasons patients come to me is pain in the area of the shoulder. Shoulder pain, both in the front and the back of the shoulder, can be due to an inflamed structure in your cervical spine, even though your neck may not hurt! Look at **Picture 195**. What you will see is that the C4-C5, the C5-C6, and the C6-C7 discs, facet joints, or nerves can create pain in the front and/or back of the shoulder.

The shoulder pain from the cervical spine can appear to be coming from the shoulder, as it is painful at times to move the shoulder, even though there is nothing wrong with the shoulder. Chapter 8 gives you more information regarding shoulder pain from the cervical spine.

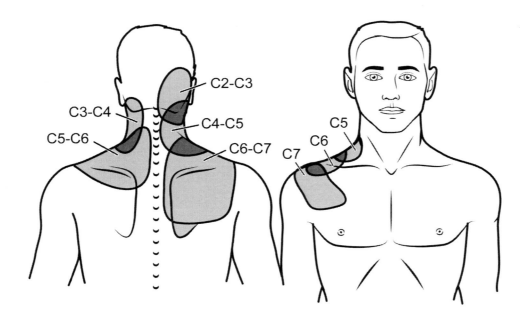

C2-C3
C3-C4
C5-C6
C4-C5
C6-C7
C5
C6
C7

PICTURE 195

Shoulder pain created by inflamed cervical discs, facet joints, and/or nerves.

8. How do I exercise if I have a problem with my back or neck?

I started the **Straight Spine Safe Spine** Program so that patients with a bad back or neck can still exercise safely, which will not only help you maintain your body weight, but also teach you proper body mechanics so that you do not re-inflame the structure that was creating your pain. For years I have had a cervical spine problem myself, so I designed this program after my own difficulties in the gym made me change how I was exercising.

Being overweight makes a difference in the way you exercise for two reasons. The weight of the body is going to create an increased level of pressure on the structures of the spine, which over time may create inflammation and pain. The other problem is that carrying excess weight makes it very difficult to maintain proper body mechanics. Trying to bend your knees and maintain a straight spine becomes exceedingly difficult as your body weight increases. Numerous patients have experienced a dramatic decrease in their pain after losing weight, and most of these patients no longer need to see me as a physician because of their new ability to exercise and maintain good posture and mechanics.

One of the differences in the **Straight Spine Safe Spine** Program, compared to most workout programs, is that it is *specific* for the problem in your spine, whether it is your neck, mid-back, or lower back. Once you know what is creating your pain, you can then do the right exercises so that you do not aggravate the underlying problem in your spine. Chapter 17 gives you information regarding body mechanics as well as exercises that you can do to strengthen your body while keeping your spine safe.

9. Why should patients wean themselves off long-term narcotic pain medications before undergoing minimally invasive procedures?

I have had very little success doing diagnostic or therapeutic minimally invasive procedures on patients with chronic spine pain when they have been taking significant amounts of narcotic pain medications for an extended period of time. The problem is the hypersensitivity to pain that occurs once people have been on narcotics for just several months to years. I have found that these patients' perception of pain is so altered by the narcotics that even if I eliminate the inflammation from the structure in the spine that is creating the pain, it is very difficult to obtain a diagnostic answer or provide any long-term relief. The question at that point is whether their pain is due to the problem in their spine or to the narcotics themselves.

If patients allow me to help them wean themselves off most of the narcotics prior to a minimally invasive procedure, two things happen. First, many patients feel much better because they are no longer hypersensitive to pain. Second, the minimally invasive procedures are significantly more successful!

10. What type of physical therapy and/or exercises do I need for my back pain?

Physical therapy should be *specific* for the problem causing your discomfort. Back pain can be due to a herniated disc, arthritic joints, or spinal stenosis, which is a condition that is created when your spinal canal narrows, and the same exercises cannot be used for all of these problems. For example, **Picture 196** shows a common physical therapy exercise for back pain where you lie on the floor and arch your back.

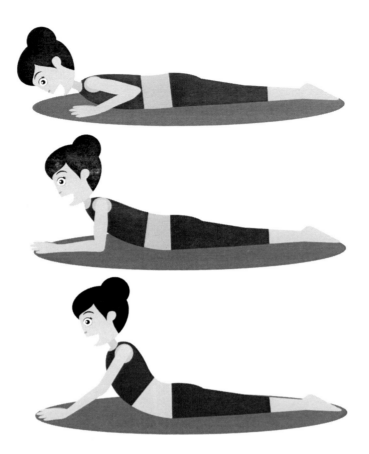

PICTURE 196

Exercise that may help push the herniated disc away from the nerve.

This is an excellent exercise if your back and/or leg pain is due to a herniated disc pressing on the nerve, as this exercise may help push the disc away from the nerve and subsequently reduce your discomfort. But if your back and/or leg pain is due to spinal stenosis, then the arching of your back while doing this exercise can narrow the spinal canal and may make your discomfort worse. You need a *specific* physical therapy and exercise program for your *specific* problem.

The **Straight Spine Safe Spine** Therapy and Exercise Program that is covered in Chapter 17 has been designed to provide *specific* exercises for your *specific* problem. The program may not only help you decrease your pain, but will also teach you proper body mechanics as well as show you how to safely strengthen your body, so that you can decrease the chances of having recurrences of your pain.

For more information on spine pain conditions and treatments and to order additional books, visit **www.straightspinesafespine.com**.